Basic Healthcare Statistics for Health Information Management Professionals

Revised Edition

Basic Healthcare Statistics for Health Information Management Professionals

Revised Edition

Karen G. Youmans, MPA, RHIA, CCS

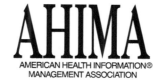

AMERICAN HEALTH INFORMATION®
MANAGEMENT ASSOCIATION

First edition 1996

ISBN 1-58426-042-4
AHIMA product No. AB120700
Production No. IPC-3000-201

American Health Information Management Association
233 North Michigan Avenue, Suite 2150
Chicago, Illinois 60601-5800

http://www.ahima.org

Contents

About the Author ix

Acknowledgments xi

Introduction xiii

Chapter 1 **Mathematics Review**. 1

   Basic Review of Ratio, Proportion, Percentage, and Rate 2

   Measures of Central Tendency. 5

Chapter 2 **Patient Census Data** 9

   Census. 10

   Daily Census. 12

   Inpatient Service Days. 13

   Total Inpatient Service Days 14

   Test on Definitions 14

   Calculation of Inpatient Service Days 16

   Assignment No. 1 20

   Test on Computation of Census and Inpatient Service Days. 21

   Average Daily Census 22

   Test on Average Daily Census 25

Chapter 3 **Bed Occupancy Ratio** 27

   Bed Count. 28

   Bed Count Days 29

   Bed Occupancy Ratio 29

   Bed Turnover Rate 32

   Test on Bed Occupancy Ratio 33

   Assignment No. 2 35

Chapter 4   **Length of Stay Data** 37
  Length of Stay 38
  Total Length of Stay 39
  Average Length of Stay 40
  Average Newborn Length of Stay 42
  Test on Length of Stay 42

Chapter 5   **Obstetrical and Perinatal Rates** 45
  Infant Mortality Rate 46
  Fetal Death Rate 48
  Maternal Death Rate 49
  Cesarean Section Rate 50
  Test on Obstetrical and Perinatal Rates 52

Chapter 6   **Morbidity and Other Rates** 53
  Infection Rate 54
  Postoperative Infection Rate 54
  Other Rates 55
  Test on Morbidity and Other Rates 58

Chapter 7   **Death (Mortality) Rates** 59
  Death Rate 60
  Other, Specific Death Rate Data 61
  Cancer Mortality Rate 62
  Test on Death (Mortality) Rates 63

Chapter 8   **Hospital Autopsies and Autopsy Rates** 65
  Gross Autopsy Rate 66
  Net Autopsy Rate 66
  Hospital Autopsies 67
  Adjusted Hospital Autopsy Rate 68
  Test on Hospital Autopsies and Autopsy Rates 69
  Test on Chapters 7 and 8 71

Chapter 9   **Statistics Computed within the Health Information
             Management Department** 73
  Staff Workload and Productivity 74
  Work Space 79

Chapter 10 **Statistics Computed for Alternative Care Settings** 83
    Managed Care Organizations. 84
    Ambulatory Care Facilities 87
    Long-Term Care Facilities. 87
    Behavioral Health Settings 90

Chapter 11 **Measures of Variation**. 93
    Variability 94
    Range 94
    Variance 95
    Standard Deviation 96
    Test on Measures of Variation 98
    Test Validation Exercise 99

Chapter 12 **Data Presentation** 101
    Types of Data 102
    Data Display 104
    Test on Data Presentation 112
    Assignment No. 3 113

Chapter 13 **Computerization of Statistics** 115
    Verification of Reports. 116
    Use of Spreadsheets. 117
    Assignment No.4. 124

References and Bibliography 127
Review Exercises. 129
Appendix A: Formulas. 135
Appendix B: Glossary of Healthcare Services and Statistical Terms. 139
Index 177

About the Author

Karen Garrett Youmans, MPA, RHIA, CCS, received her associate degree from Sinclair Community College in Dayton, Ohio; her bachelor's degree in health information administration from the College of St. Scholastica in Duluth, Minnesota; and her master's in public administration, health services management major, from Golden Gate University, MacDill Air Force Base, in Tampa, Florida.

Currently a practice manager for the coding products and services team for AHIMA, Karen works from her home. Previously, she was a client resource specialist with CodeMaster of Santa Cruz, California. In addition, she was an assistant professor in the health information management program at the University of Central Florida, in Orlando, and program director of medical record technology at St. Petersburg Junior College in St. Petersburg, Florida. She has taught many seminars for the Central Florida HIMA, the Gulf Coast Florida HIMA, and the Florida HIMA.

Karen has volunteered her services in many capacities for both AHIMA and the Florida HIMA (FHIMA). She served on the AHIMA Board of Directors from 1995–1997 and, before that, served as chair of the Council on Accreditation and a director on the Assembly on Education Board. She also has served as president of FHIMA and on numerous committees on the state level. For her efforts, she received FHIMA's Distinguished Member Award and its Literary Award.

In addition to contributing numerous articles to the *Journal of AHIMA,* she has served four times as guest editor. She also was project manager and coeditor of the 1992 revision of the *Florida Medical/Legal Guide,* and authored a chapter on methods for analyzing and improving systems in *Health Information: Management of a Strategic Resource,* published by W. B. Saunders Company.

She currently lives in Lawrenceville, Georgia, with her husband, Walt, and her children, Nick and Vanessa.

Acknowledgments

The staff of the American Health Information Management Association and author Karen Youmans extend deepest gratitude to glossary writer Barbara Glondys. Due to an editorial oversight, her name was not included in the initial printing of this edition. We apologize to Ms. Glondys and thank her for her invaluable contribution to this book.

The author wishes to thank Carol Barr, Kathy Cameron, Janice Copeland, Claire Dixon-Lee, Michelle Dougherty, Rose Dunn, Vi Griffin, Carole Howard, Lynn Kuehn, Janice Leybold, Desla Mancilla, Ruby Nicholson, Bryon Pickard, Pam Rollins, Judy Smith, and Sue Watkins, whose ideas and statistical information helped form the case studies included in this text. Additional thanks to the students at the University of Central Florida in Orlando.

The AHIMA staff would also like to thank the reviewers of this book for their insightful comments and suggestions.

The author dedicates this text to Walt, Nick, Vanessa, and Imogene, and the memory of Cecil H. Garrett and Patricia J. Pierce.

Introduction

The field of statistics may be defined as the science and art of gathering, analyzing, and interpreting data. Facts set down as numbers, statistics enable information to be extracted from a mass of raw data. To serve their purpose, the figures must be relevant and reliable.

In healthcare, the primary source of data used in compiling statistics is the health record. Healthcare statistics have many uses. For example, a physical therapy department may use statistical information such as the number of patient visits in deciding whether to hire additional physical therapists. Indeed, many states use statistics when they issue hospital "report cards." These state report cards, which are available to the public and published in local newspapers, compare hospitals' death rates, lengths of stay, readmission rates, average charges, and percentages of births requiring cesarean sections.

Because health information management (HIM) practitioners have a broad knowledge of healthcare facilities as well as immediate access to a wide range of clinical data, they are in the best position to collect, prepare, analyze, and interpret healthcare data. HIM practitioners must learn acceptable terminology, definitions, and computational methodology if they are to provide the basic and most frequently used health statistics. To that end, this book is designed to introduce statistical computation at the introductory level for use in health information technician (HIT) or health information administration (HIA) educational programs.

Although intended primarily for students just beginning their health statistics course, this book also can be used by any health professional interested in acquiring knowledge and ability in this area. Moreover, it can be used, in part, in the assessment of students transferring from a two-year HIT program to a four-year HIA program. Further, it can be used with independent study materials by students wishing to advance more rapidly through the required sequence as well as by students needing additional assistance. Finally, it can be used as a reference or continuing educational tool for the experienced HIM practitioner.

Guidelines for Using This Book

HIM practitioners may be asked to produce an almost limitless number of rates from data collection. However, as an introduction to the field, this book discusses only on those healthcare statistics that HIM professionals compute most often. Moreover, it focuses on commonly used rates and percentages computed principally on hospital inpatients. However, the author also has included non-acute care data and examples. Therefore, when a definition or formula states *patient,* it also could mean *client, member,* or *resident.*

Although *Basic Healthcare Statistics for Health Information Management Professionals* examines definitions and formulas found in various references, it relies most heavily on those contained in Appendix B: *Glossary of Healthcare Services and Statistical Terms.* (The glossary, which was originally available from AHIMA as a separate publication, is also designed as a useful reference beyond the classroom.) It is expected that you will be able to determine logically any rate that you are requested to determine.

Finally, throughout this book, a number of figures and tables display actual, unaltered statistical reports from the "real world" of health information management. Their inclusion in the book has a specific purpose. The so-called real world sometimes produces mistaken or misleading information. For example, a facility may not follow the rules as stated in this book for creating tables or rounding to the correct decimal. Therefore, the "actual reports" included in a number of exercises are included to challenge students and other readers to find and validate or correct the errors they contain.

Chapter 1
Mathematics Review

Objectives

At the conclusion of this chapter, you should be able to:

- Convert fractions to percentages
- Differentiate among ratio, proportion, percentage, and rate
- Define and compute mean, median, and mode

Basic Review of Ratio, Proportion, Percentage, and Rate

The term *rate* is often used loosely to refer to rate, proportion, percentage, and ratio. Indeed, many books and organizations use these terms interchangeably. For this reason, it is important to be aware of how any measure being reported has actually been defined and calculated.

Calculating Rate

The basic rule of thumb for calculating rate is to indicate the number of times that something actually happened in relation to the number of times that something could have happened $^{(actual}/_{potential)}$ For example, your everyday life has been hectic the past few weeks, and according to your bathroom scale (and your wallet), you have been eating out too often. To calculate the rate of meals eaten out, divide the number of times you have eaten out per week (for example, 13) by the number of meals in a week that you could have eaten out (21). The rate would be 61.9 percent, or $^{13}/_{21}$.

The health information management (HIM) practitioner may calculate ratios, proportions, percentages, and/or rates; interpret computer output; or validate data reports. Data may be reported to various state agencies. Examples of data reported by HIM professionals include:

- In Florida, patient discharge data are submitted electronically to the Agency for Health Care Administration (AHCA), which compares hospitals' death rates, lengths of stay, readmission rates, average charges, and percentage of births requiring cesarean sections.

- Data submitted to AHCA for 1997 indicated that Medicare accounted for 41.9 percent of total discharges, with a mean LOS of 6.1; commercial patients represented 33.2 percent of all discharges, with a mean LOS of 4.0.

- A report published by the Colorado State Inpatient Database showed that for discharges in 1997, the number one reason for hospitalization was live borns, with pneumonia placing second.

- The U.S. Agency for Healthcare Research and Quality (AHRQ) has recently made public its HCUPnet—a free, interactive online service that allows people to look up data compiled from seven million patients at 1,000 hospitals in twenty-two states. With HCUPnet, you have easy access to national and selected state statistics about hospital stays.

Everyday examples of rates that HIM practitioners encounter include percentage of bed occupancy, admission rates, death rates, and percentage of Medicare patients. Table 1.1 shows an actual report.

Calculating Ratio

Three general classes of mathematical parameters are used to relate the number of cases, diseases, patients, or outcomes in the healthcare environment to the size of the source population in which they occur. The most basic measure is the ratio. Ratio is calculated by dividing one quantity by another. For example, if six men and 10 women were in a group,

Table 1.1.   Percent of Revenue by Payer Type

Community Hospital
Percent of Revenue by Payer Type
Inpatient and Outpatient

	This Month				This Year		
Payer	**Inpatient**	**Outpatient**	**Total**	**Payer**	**Inpatient**	**Outpatient**	**Total**
Medicare	74.0%	42.4%	61.5%	Medicare	72.4%	4.1%	62.2%
Medicaid	1.6%	3.8%	2.5%	Medicaid	2.0%	3.1%	2.4%
Commercial	15.0%	31.2%	21.4%	Commercial	17.8%	31.7%	22.8%
Blue Cross	5.7%	7.6%	6.4%	Blue Cross	3.3%	8.2%	5.1%
HMO	1.7%	6.2%	3.5%	HMO	2.0%	7.2%	3.9%
Other	2.0%	8.8%	4.7%	Other	2.5%	5.7%	3.6%
Total	**100.0%**	**100.0%**	**100.0%**	**Total**	**100.0%**	**100.0%**	**100.0%**

the ratio of men to women would be $^6/_{10}$. The number can be greater than 1 or less than 1 *Ratio* is a general term that can include a number of specific measures such as proportion, percentage, and rate (Hennekens and Buring 1987).

$$\textbf{Ratio: } \frac{a}{b} = \frac{1}{12}$$

or

$$\textbf{Ratio: } \frac{b}{a} = \frac{12}{1}$$

Proportion as a Type of Ratio

A *proportion* is a type of ratio in which the elements included in the numerator (the top number) also must be included in the denominator (the bottom number). For example, if two women out of a group of ten over the age of 50 have had ovarian cancer, the proportion would be written as 2:10, 2 in 10, or $^2/_{10}$.

$$\textbf{Proporation: } \frac{a}{(a + b)} = \frac{2}{(2 + 8)}$$

Percentage as a Type of Ratio

The ratio of a part to the whole is often expressed as a *percentage*. Percentage is computed on the basis of the whole divided into 100 parts. It is a specific way to write a fraction (for example, $^1/_{10} = 10\%$). The quotient is the result of 10 dividing one number by another. A quotient is converted to a percent by multiplying the quotient by 100 or moving the decimal point two spaces to the right (Hennekens and Buring 1987).

$$\text{Example: } \frac{\text{numerator}}{\text{denominator}} \rightarrow \frac{1}{4} = .25 \times 100 = 25\%$$

Not all percentages are converted to whole numbers, for example:

$$\frac{1}{8} = .125 = 12.5\%$$

Each healthcare facility has its own policy on the number of decimal places used in computing and reporting percentages. The division process then should be carried out to one more place in the quotient and rounded back. For example:

$$\frac{1}{7} = .14285 = 14.285\% = 14.29\%$$

The general rule for rounding is to drop the last figure if it is less than 5 and to add one unit to the preceding figure if the last figure is 5 or more. For example, 14.285 is rounded to 14.29; 14.284 is rounded to 14.28.

Rate as a Type of Ratio

A *rate* is a ratio in which there is a distinct relationship between numerator and denominator and the denominator often implies a large base population. A measure of time is often an intrinsic part of the denominator. For example, rates could include the number of newly diagnosed cases of breast cancer per 100,000 women in a particular year, the number of cases of head lice per 1,000 elementary school students in a one-month period, or the number of deaths in a year at a particular hospital (Hennekens and Buring 1987).

Careful attention should be given to rates and percentages. Mathematical errors can occur due to misplaced decimal points. All calculations should be checked for sense. For example, a death rate of 25 percent should seem unreasonable. Would you want to be treated at a hospital that had a 25 percent death rate? That would mean one of every four patients treated at that hospital dies. Check the calculation as well as the decimal placement. For example, the death rate may be 2.5 percent or .25 percent.

The following example differentiates among ratio, proportion, percentage, and rate:

$$a = men;\ b = women$$

Ratio: $\dfrac{a}{b}$

Proportion: $\dfrac{a}{(a + b)}$

Percentage: $\left[\dfrac{a}{(a + b)}\right] \times 100$

Rate: $\left[\dfrac{a}{(a + b)}\right] \times 100$ *for a specific period of time, or for a large-based population*

Table 1.2 shows an actual computerized statistical report provided by the information systems department of an acute care facility.

Everyone has heard this saying about computers: "garbage in, garbage out." Computers are great for many things, including performing statistical calculations, but they must be programmed accurately to calculate correctly. Even the function of rounding needs to be validated. For example, it is not unheard of for an information systems manager to ask an HIM professional for the formula for death rate because the computer system crashed and all new formulas and specifications had to be programmed again.

More examples of computerized statistical reports are given throughout this book. It is important to keep in mind that basic competence in mathematics is an essential element in the practice of health information management.

Table 1.2.   Administrator's Semiannual Reference Report

Admissions by Day of Week
1/1/99–6/30/99

Day	Number of Patients	Percent of Patients
Sunday	1,187	17.9
Monday	755	11.3
Tuesday	1,085	16.3
Wednesday	1,031	15.5
Thursday	1,024	15.3
Friday	808	12.1
Saturday	773	11.6
Total	**6,663**	**100.0**

Exercise 1.1

1. Convert the fraction $^1/_5$ to quotient and then to a percentage.

2. Round the following percentages to two places past the decimal point.

    A. 14.3690%
    B. 29.896%
    C. 0.565%
    D. 0.055%
    E. 78.65432%

3. Using the general rule of reporting percentages to two places past the decimal point, convert $^1/_6$ to a percentage.

4. Review table 1.2 to verify that the calculations are correct. Note that the percent of patients listed in this report is the actual/potential.

$$\left(\frac{Actual\ \#\ of\ patients}{Potential\ \#\ of\ patients} \right) \times 100$$

Measures of Central Tendency

In summarizing data, it is often useful to have a single *typical* or *average* number that is representative of the entire collection of data or specific population. Such numbers are customarily referred to as *measures of central tendency.* Everyone is familiar with some type of average. For example, you can compare your weight to that of a typical person on a weight chart. Students are familiar with their own average in a given course. One of the most common examples of averaging in the healthcare arena is length of stay, or LOS (number of days from admission to discharge that a patient stays in the hospital). Average length of stay is discussed briefly in this chapter and in detail in chapter 4.

Three measures of central tendency are frequently used: mean, median, and mode. Each measure has advantages and disadvantages in describing a typical value.

Mean

The *mean* is the arithmetic average. It is common to use the term *average* to designate mean. To obtain the mean, add all the values in a frequency distribution and then divide the total by the number of values in the distribution.

> Example: Seven hospital inpatients have the following lengths of stay: 2, 3, 4, 3, 5, 1, 3. The total of all the values is 21. When the total is divided by the number of values involved (7), the average length of stay, or mean ($\bar{x}$), is equal to three days.

The symbol $\bar{x}$ (pronounced X bar) is used to represent the mean (Hennekens and Buring 1987).

$$\textbf{Mean Formula: } \frac{\textit{Total of all the values (sum)}}{\textit{Number of the values involved}} = \bar{x}$$

The mean is the most common measure of central tendency. It is used as a basis for a large proportion of statistical tests. However, the mean is not sensitive to extreme values (called *outliers*) that may distort its representation of the typical value of a set of numbers. For example, if six women in a group weighed 110, 115, 120, 122, 125, and 227 pounds, the mean weight of the group would be $819/6$, or 136.5 pounds. However, given that five of the women weigh 125 pounds or less, the mean of this sample is not a good indication of a typical observation. Thus, the more asymmetric or unequal the distribution, the less desirable it is to summarize the observations by using the mean.

Median

The *median* is the midpoint (center) of the distribution of values. It is the point above and below which 50 percent of the values lies. The median describes the literal middle of the data. The median value is obtained by arranging the numerical observations in ascending or descending order and then determining the value in the middle of the array. This may be the middle observation (if there is an odd number of values) or a point halfway between the two middle values (if there is an even number of values).

Using the LOS example above, the numbers are sequenced as:

1

2

3

3 ← median (midpoint)

3

4

5

The median is 3.

The median weight of the women who weighed 110, 115, 120, 122, 125, and 227 pounds is shown as:

110
115
120 ← median $(120 + 122 = \dfrac{242}{2} = 121)$
122
125
227
The median is 121.

The advantage to the median as a measure of central tendency is that it is unaffected by extreme values. The value of 121 is much more representative of the fact that five out of the six women weigh 125 pounds or less than the mean value of 136.5. The disadvantage is that because its value is determined solely by rank, it provides no information about any of the other values within the distribution (Hennekens and Buring 1987).

Mode

The *mode* is the most recurring or most frequent value in a given set of data. It is rarely used as a sole descriptive measure of central tendency. In the case of a small number of values, each value likely occurs only once and there may be no mode. Again, referring to the LOS example, the mode would be 3 because 3 is the most frequent value in the set. Sometimes examination of the mode can provide insights into the possible etiology of a disease process. For example, an observation of a frequency distribution of age at diagnosis of Hodgkin's disease yielded two modes: age 29 and age 73 (Hennekens and Buring 1987).

The choice of a measure of central tendency depends on the number of values and the nature of their distribution. Sometimes the mean, median, and mode are identical, as in the LOS example above. For statistical analyses, however, the mean is preferable, whenever possible, because it includes information from all observations. But if the data are asymmetric or skewed, the median may need to be considered. When the series of values contains a few that are unusually high, the median may represent the series better than the mean. The mode is often used in samples where the data are not numerical. For example, if students were asked to select the *typical* student from among 10 candidates, the one with the most votes (mode) would be selected (Hennekens and Buring 1987).

Add another patient's length of stay (35) to the previous example. The values would now total 56 (1 + 2 + 3 + 3 + 3 + 4 + 5 + 35). Divide 56 by the number of values involved (8) to calculate the mean of 7, or $^{56}/_8 = 7$

The median would be calculated as follows:
1
2
3
3 ←median $(3 + 3 = \dfrac{6}{2} = 3)$
3
4
5
35
The median is 3.

This example shows that the median is unaffected by extreme values.

Exercise 1.2

1. Fourteen patients have the following lengths of stay: 2, 3, 4, 1, 4, 16, 4, 2, 1, 5, 4, 3, 6, 1. Compute the mean, median, and mode.

2. A student's scores on ten 10-point class quizzes include a 5, a 7, an 8, six 9s, and a 10. The student claims that her average grade on quizzes is 9 because most of her scores are 9s. Is this correct? Explain.

For the following questions, refer to the transcription accuracy report below.

3. Check the calculation of the monthly averages for October. Is the calculation correct?

4. Transcriptionist H has a year-to-date accuracy rate of 98.9 percent. She would like you to recalculate her accuracy rate because she thinks it is incorrect.

Memorial Health System
Transcription Accuracy

Fiscal Year 1999

Transcriptionist	Oct	Nov	Dec	Jan	Feb	Mar	Apr	May	June	July	Aug	Sept	FY99 AVG YTD
A	94.8	98	97.3	97	97.2	97.7	97.7	97.6	99	98.1			97.4
B	98	99	97	98.5	98.3	97.4	96	98	96.4	98.1			97.7
C	98.3	98.3	99.9	98.6	99.3	100	99.4	98.8	98.5	98.7			99.0
D	98.2	98.6	97.7	98	99.3	98.7	99.1	99	97.7	98.3			98.5
E	98.2	99.9	99.2	99.3	98.2	99.2	98.8	99.4	98.2	98.3			98.9
F	99.2	100	99.3	99.3	99.8	98.3	98.2	99.6	100	99.1			99.3
G	98.7	99.6	99.8	99.8	99.6	98.6	97	97.3	98.3	99			98.8
H	100	96.2	100	99.3	98.2	99.6	98.2	99.6	99.3	99			98.9
I	98.9	99.2	98	100	99.8	98.8	LOA	0	0	0			99.1
J	0	0	0	0	0	0	0	0	0	99.3			99.3
K	97.5	98.4	99.4	98	97.4	98.4	97.8	98.4	98.4	98			98.2
L	0	0	0	0	0	0	0	0	0	98.4			98.4
M	100	99.3	98.9	99.5	98.8	100	99.4	99.7	0	0			99.5
N	100	98	97.5	98	98.1	98.6	100	99.4	98.4	98.1			98.4
O	98.2	99.9	99.3	99	100	98.2	98.4	99.3	99.7	99.8			99.1
P	99.3	99	98.2	99	98.2	98.1	99	98.5	99.1	98			98.6
Q	0	0	0	99.2	0	0	0	0	0	0			99.2
R	98.9	99.2	93	98.1	98.4	97.7	98.9	97.4	99.6	98			97.6
Monthly Averages	**98.54**	**98.84**	**98.3**	**98.78**	**98.70**	**98.62**	**98.42**	**98.71**	**98.66**	**98.54**	**0**	**0**	**98.7**

Chapter 2
Patient Census Data

Objectives

At the conclusion of this chapter, you should be able to:

- Define, differentiate, and apply the terms *census, daily census, inpatient service day,* and *total inpatient service days*
- Compute daily census and inpatient service days using admission and discharge data provided
- Compute census and inpatient service days with data given for births and transfers
- Compute average daily census for a patient care unit given inpatient service days for any such unit

Census

The *census* indicates the number of patients present in the healthcare facility at any given time. Hospitals will only include inpatients in their calculations. Management uses census data for various purposes, including planning, budgeting, and staffing. An individual on each patient care unit (PCU) is designated to count the patients on that unit daily. The inpatient census-taking time is usually at midnight (12 A.M.) but may occur at any time as long as the time is adhered to consistently.

In a manual system, the census taker fills out a form to be sent to a central collection area (usually the nursing office, data processing/information systems, or health information). The names of patients admitted, discharged, and transferred to or from a PCU are included on the form. This makes it easier for the central collection area to discover any discrepancies in the data from the PCUs and to know where each patient is located at all times.

In a computerized system, the necessary data are first entered into the computer as admissions, discharges, or transfers and then verified at the designated time by the responsible person on each PCU. Table 2.1 shows an actual manual daily midnight census summary for a nursing home.

Census Data Used to Calculate Staffing Hours

As mentioned earlier, management sometimes uses census data for staffing purposes. Table 2.2 is an actual report showing an analysis of daily staffing hours at a nursing home. Every state-licensing agency has specific guidelines or requirements for staffing. In table 2.2, the staffing required for each patient needing a skilled staff member is 2.6 hours and the staffing required for the remaining patients is 2.35 hours.

The calculation used to determine staffing hours is as follows:

*Number of nurses × 8 hours + number of nursing assistants × 7.5 hours
+ other hours = the total*

The total number of required staffing hours then is compared to the total number of hours provided by the staff. This nursing home calculates staffing on a daily basis to analyze whether it is under- or overstaffed and within state requirements. On day one, the required staffing hours were 307.15, but the nursing home provided only 302.75 staffing hours. Thus, the facility was understaffed by 4.4 hours. On day two, it was understaffed by 17.4 hours. So the facility's accumulated total for days one and two is 21.8 hours understaffed. The census is key to this analysis.

Complete Master Census

In addition to reporting the head count to the central collection area, each PCU also reports, either in written form or via computer, the number of patients admitted, discharged, and/or transferred in or out that day. The central collection area then uses the census from all the units to compile a total census for the hospital, sometimes referred to as the *complete master census*. The complete master census shows the number of patients present in the hospital at any given time.

In this book, the term *transfer* in a hospital setting refers to an intrahospital transfer. *Intrahospital transfers* are patients transferred from one PCU to another within the facility. Admission, discharge, and transfer data are used throughout the program.

Table 2.1. **Daily Midnight Census Summary at XYZ Nursing Home**

XYZ MANOR NURSING HOME
Daily Midnight Census Summary

To be completed daily at
midnight by charge nurse

Hall: | A | B | C | D |

Date

Initial admits—New residents		Date	Time
			AM–PM
			AM–PM
			AM–PM
			AM–PM
Discharged—To home or transfer		Date	Time
			AM–PM
			AM–PM
			AM–PM
Transfer to hospital	Location	Date	Time
			AM–PM
			AM–PM
			AM–PM
			AM–PM

Out on leave—Pass	Date Left	Time	Returned	Time
		AM–PM		AM–PM
		AM–PM		AM–PM
		AM–PM		AM–PM

Deceased		Date	Time of Death
			AM–PM
			AM–PM
			AM–PM
Return from hospital stay		Date	Time
			AM–PM
			AM–PM
			AM–PM
			AM–PM

Charge nurse: _____

Table 2.2. **Chart Analysis of Staffing Hours at XYZ Nursing Home**

XYZ MANOR NURSING HOME
DAILY STAFFING—HOURS ANALYSIS

Date

Date	1	2	3	4	5	6	7	8	9	10	11	12
Census	129	129	129	129	130	129	129	129	129	128	128	129
Skilled	16	16	16	16	16	15	15	15	15	14	14	14
NFs	113	113	113	113	114	114	114	114	114	114	114	115
Total												
Req. hours	307.15	307.15	307.15	307.15	309.5	306.9	306.9	306.9	306.9	304.3	304.3	306.65
Staffing												
Nurses	7	5	4	7	7	7	8	7	5	5	8	5
Nursing assts.	30	26	28	26	31	31	30	19	32	33	32	32
Other & OT (# hrs.)	21.75	54.75	63.25	47.75	31	36.25	46.25	119.25	28	28.25	46 28	
Total Hrs. provided	302.75	289.75	305.25	298.75	319.5	324.75	319.25	317.75	308	315.75	350	308
Summary												
Daily +/−	−4.4	−17.4	−1.9	−8.4	10	17.85	12.35	10.85	1.1	11.45	45.7	1.35
(1st thru 15th) Accum. Total	−4.4	−21.8	−23.7	−32.1	−22.1	−4.25	8.1	18.95	20.05	31.5	77.2	78.55

Exercise 2.1

1. Unit A has a count of 20 patients at 1 A.M. on June 1 and 30 patients at the same time on June 2. Could the counts have been different if unit A had taken a census at midnight on both days?

2. Would you accept the different patient care units in the hospital taking censuses at different times as long as each unit is consistent within itself?

3. A patient transferred at 5 P.M. to unit A from unit B is counted in unit A's midnight census as one additional patient present. Would that patient still be included in unit B's midnight census?

Daily Census

The *daily census* includes the number of inpatients present on the PCU at the census-taking time each day and any inpatients who were both admitted after the previous census-taking time and discharged before the next census-taking time. Thus, a patient admitted to the PCU at 8 A.M. on June 1 and discharged at 10 P.M. that same day would not be present for the PCU's midnight head count. However, because the patient must be accounted for in some manner, he or she is included in the unit's midnight census.

Exercise 2.2

1. The daily census at 12 A.M. on May 31 is 100. The new 24-hour period begins at 12:01 A.M. Two patients are admitted on June 1 at 7 A.M. and discharged at approximately 8 P.M. that same day. One patient is admitted at 1 P.M. but dies at 4:30 P.M. the same afternoon. What is the PCU's daily census for June 1?

2. Which would be the better form of data to keep permanently, census or daily census? Why?

Inpatient Service Days

An *inpatient service day* is a unit of measure denoting the services received by one inpatient in one 24-hour period. The 24-hour period is the time between the census-taking hours on two successive days. When the census-taking time is midnight, a 24-hour period is the same as the calendar day (that is, from 12:01 A.M. through 12 P.M.). One inpatient service day is counted for each inpatient admission where a patient is admitted and discharged the same day (that is, between two successive census-taking hours). If this is not done, credit for the services rendered to that patient is lost.

A number of important conventions concerning inpatient service days are listed in Appendix B: *Glossary of Healthcare Services and Statistical Terms,* and *Health Information Management* (Huffman 1994). These conventions include:

-   One unit of one service day is not usually divided or reported as a fraction of a day.

-   The day of admission is counted as an inpatient service day, but the day of discharge is not.

-   The days a patient does not occupy a bed due to leave of absence are excluded because he or she is not present at the census-taking hour. An absence of less than one day is not considered a leave of absence in compiling statistics. A physician may authorize a leave of absence for a patient for various reasons, including a holiday, a family wedding, or a funeral. When the patient or physician believes the advantages of an absence from the facility outweigh the advantages of uninterrupted hospitalization, the hospital has the choice of discharging and then readmitting the patient or granting a leave of absence.

Inpatient service day is the correct term to use for what is commonly referred to as a *patient day, inpatient day, bed occupancy day,* or *census day.* The correct wording reflects the hospital function of providing services to patients each day. If twenty patients are provided services in one 24-hour period, the number of inpatient service days for that calendar day is twenty.

Exercise 2.3

Compare the definition of inpatient service day to the definitions of daily census and census. Will the figure representing inpatient service day for any one day be the same as the figure for daily census or census?

Total Inpatient Service Days

The term *total inpatient service days* refers to the sum of all the inpatient service days in the period under consideration. For example, if the inpatient service days for June 1, 2, and 3 are 100, 105, and 101, the total for the three days is 306. Typically, total inpatient service days are calculated monthly, quarterly, semiannually, or annually.

Exercise 2.4

Given the following inpatient service days for a 65-bed hospital, what is the total number of inpatient service days provided in June?

June 1: 50	June 11: 48	June 21: 55
2: 50	12: 56	22: 58
3: 49	13: 58	23: 62
4: 54	14: 56	24: 65
5: 52	15: 59	25: 63
6: 51	16: 60	26: 62
7: 50	17: 59	27: 60
8: 43	18: 58	28: 60
9: 44	19: 54	29: 62
10: 46	20: 55	30: 63

Test on Definitions

Select the best answer to each of the following questions:

1. The difference between a census and a daily census is that any patients admitted and discharged the same day are added to:

    a. The census to compute the daily census
    b. The midnight (or other designated time) head count to compute the daily census
    c. Both a and b
    d. None of the above

2. Because they are a unit of measure, the data used for most census computations are:

   a. The census
   b. The daily census
   c. Total inpatient service days
   d. None of the above

3. The time for taking the inpatient census must always be:

   a. Midnight
   b. Consistent
   c. 12:00 P.M.
   d. 11:59 P.M.

4. At census-taking time, a patient who has been transferred into a unit is

   a. Counted where he or she is
   b. Counted where he or she came from
   c. Not counted
   d. Counted in both units

5. Patient day or inpatient day is more correctly termed:

   a. Inpatient service day
   b. Daily inpatient census
   c. Total inpatient service day(s)
   d. Census

6. To calculate the total inpatient service days for a period, add:

   a. All inpatient service days for the period
   b. The inpatient census for the period
   c. The daily inpatient census for the period
   d. Any of the above

7. The inpatient census at midnight is 50. One patient was admitted at 1 P.M. and died at 3:15 P.M. The inpatient service days for that day are:

   a. 49
   b. 50
   c. 51
   d. None of the above

8. Define the following terms:

   a. Census
   b. Daily census
   c. Inpatient service day
   d. Total inpatient service days

Calculation of Inpatient Service Days

The calculation of inpatient service days is the measurement of services received by all inpatients in one 24-hour period (the time between the census-taking hours on two successive days). Thus, when the census-taking time is midnight, the 24-hour period is 12 A.M. through 11:59 P.M. In addition, one inpatient day must be counted for each inpatient admitted and discharged the same day between two successive census-taking hours.

Sample Inpatient Service Days Display

Number of patients in hospital at 12 A.M. on October 1	250
Plus the number of patients admitted October	+ 45
Subtotal	295
Minus the number of patients discharged (including deaths) October 1	− 40
Number of patients in hospital at 11:59 P.M. on October 1 (subtotal)	255
Plus the number of patients both admitted and discharged on October 1	+ 2
Total inpatient service days for October 1	**257**

The definitions of census, inpatient service day, and total inpatient service days provide clues for actual computation. The sample above includes all of a hospital's inpatient care units. A summary of all such units helps the administration review the hospital's overall level of activity.

However, it is often necessary to exclude and study separately certain PCUs such as the newborn nursery, intensive care units (ICUs), and obstetrical units because the intensity of service on these units varies greatly from that on medical/surgical units. Hospitals may use inpatient service days to track trends from month to month or year to date.

Table 2.3 shows an actual example taken from an acute care hospital whose administration used it as a performance report.

Table 2.3. Year-to-Date Inpatient Service Days

XYZ Medical Center
April, 1995

	Actual	Budget	Prior Year
Med/Surg	12,248	12,533	14,097
Critical Care	1,149	1,209	1,293
Stepdown	897	975	1,003
Rehab	1,707	2,189	2,328
OB	1,480	1,512	1,590
Psychiatry	1,861	1,905	1,906
Neonatal ICU	948	899	916
Pediatrics	528	400	483
Total	**20,818**	**21,622**	**23,616**

XYZ medical center's analysis of its inpatient service days revealed a decline from the budget as well as a significant decrease from the prior year. This led to an examination of how the center marketed its rehabilitation services. Later, the center also analyzed the trend of healthcare from inpatient to outpatient services.

Before beginning the actual calculation of census data and inpatient service days, you should know the term *calculation of transfers*. The calculation of transfers occurs on the PCU census. Transfers in and out of the unit are shown as subdivisions of patients admitted to and discharged from the unit.

Following are some sample figures listed in a format frequently used by the central collection area:

A head count at 12 A.M. on June 1 shows 48 adult and children inpatients and two newborns. Using this starting point, take the adults and children (48) and add the number of admissions (2) and transfers in (1) to arrive at a total of 51.

(Note: Below, *a/d* indicates admitted and discharged the same day; *adm*, admissions; *b*, births; *dis*, discharges; *inpt*, inpatients; *Nb*, newborns; *A/C*, adults and children; *serv*, service; and *trf*, transfer.)

| | 12:00 census | | adm | | trf | total | | dis | Nb | trf | 11:59 census | | | serv days | |
Day	A/C	Nb	A/C	b	in	A/C	Nb	A/C	dis	out	A/C	Nb	a/d	A/C	Nb
6/1	48	2	2	1	1	51	3	1	2	1	49	1	1	50	1

Take the newborns present at 12 A.M. (2) and add the births (1) to arrive at a total of three.

| | 12:00 census | | adm | | trf | total | | dis | Nb | trf | 11:59 census | | | serv days | |
Day	A/C	Nb	A/C	b	in	A/C	Nb	A/C	dis	out	A/C	Nb	a/d	A/C	Nb
6/1	48	2	2	1	1	51	3	1	2	1	49	1	1	50	1

Next take the adults and children (51) and subtract the discharges (1) as well as the transfers out (1) for an 11:59 P.M. census of 49.

| | 12:00 census | | adm | | trf | total | | dis | Nb | trf | 11:59 census | | | serv days | |
Day	A/C	Mb	A/C	b	in	A/C	Mb	A/C	dis	out	A/C	Nb	a/d	A/C	Nb
6/1	48	2	2	1	1	51	3	1	2	1	49	1	1	50	1

Following the same procedure, take the total number of newborns (3) and subtract the newborns that were discharged (2) for an 11:59 P.M. census of one.

| | 12:00 census | | adm | | trf | total | | dis | Nb | trf | 11:59 census | | | serv days | |
Day	A/C	Nb	A/C	b	in	A/C	Nb	A/C	dis	out	A/C	Nb	a/d	A/C	Nb
6/1	48	2	2	1	1	51	3	1	2	1	49	1	1	50	1

The last two columns are discussed later in this chapter. The following points should resolve any confusion:

- *Transfers in* and *transfers out* refer to intrahospital transfers, which are transfers within the hospital. Transfers in and out of the hospital (called *interfacility transfers*) are included in admissions and discharges.

- Transfers in and out of any specific medical care unit may or may not be equal, but they must be equal for the overall hospital capitulation. Every patient transferred into a unit on any given day has to have been transferred out of another unit. Failure of these data to balance may mean that a unit neglected to report transfers correctly. It is essential that someone in the central collection area identify the source of error.

- The data of 49 adults and children and one newborn (the inpatient census at 11:59 P.M. on June 1) must be the same as the actual head count. If they are not the same, a unit may have reported admissions, discharges, or births incorrectly. Again, someone in the central collection area is responsible for finding the error.

- Newborns are considered separately for all computations based on census data. They should be reported separately unless otherwise directed by administration, medical staff, or other persons using the statistical data you produce. Births are considered newborn admissions. Services provided to newborns differ in intensity from the rest of the hospital inpatients.

- The 11:59 P.M. census at the close of one day is the inpatient census at the beginning of the next day and is commonly referred to as *number of patients remaining*.

Patients Admitted and Discharged on the Same Day

Going back to the last two columns from the previous problem, the number of patients who were admitted and discharged on the same day (a/d) must be added to the 11:59 P.M. census to show that they received services. As discussed previously, patients who are not present at either of two successive head-counting times still must be accounted for and credited with a day's care. (A patient admitted and discharged on the same day may be referred to as *in and out* (I&O) or any number of other terms or abbreviations.)

Now add the number of patients admitted and discharged on the same day (a/d) to the 11:59 P.M. census data to compute inpatient service days. Note the 50 and 1 in the last column for June 1.

Remember to begin the next day with the 11:59 P.M. census data and not inpatient service days. Calculate under the assumption that the patients admitted and discharged on the same day and the transfers are not newborns.

Recapitulation of Census Data

The process of verifying the data obtained by the process described above is called the monthly or yearly recapitulation of census data. The total number of patients admitted and born during the month or year is added to the patients-remaining census with which the month or year began. From this sum, the number of discharges during the month or year (including deaths) is subtracted. The resulting data are the number of patients remaining at

Table 2.4.   Sample Monthly Census Recapitulation

	Adults and Children	Newborns
Number of patients in hospital at 12:00 A.M. on May 1	48	2
Add the number of patients admitted in May	+ 100	+ 7
Subtotal	**148**	**− 9**
Subtract the number of patients discharged (including deaths) in May	− 110	5
Number of patients in hospital at 11:59 P.M., May 31	**38**	**4**

the end of the month or year. This should equal the actual head count at midnight of the last night of that month or year. Table 2.4 shows a sample monthly census recapitulation.

Recap is the abbreviation for recapitulation, which means to summarize. When you recap monthly (or annual) census data, you are verifying that the columns have been added correctly. This procedure also verifies that no error was made in the original data on one or more lines. This is accomplished by taking the midnight inpatient census at the beginning of the period, adding total admissions and transfers in, and subtracting total discharges and transfers out. The resultant data represent the midnight census on the last day of the period (month or year).

Exercise 2.5

1. Using the data given previously, calculate the census for June 2. With the data supplied below, how would you fill in the blanks? Also, did the transfers in and transfers out balance?

Day	12:00 census A/C	Nb	adm A/C	b	trf in	total A/C	Nb	dis A/C	Nb dis	trf out	11:59 census A/C	Nb	a/d	serv days A/C	Nb
6/1	48	2	2	1	1	51	3	1	2	1	49	1			
6/2			3	1	2			4	1	2					

2. With what data will you begin June 3, and why?

3. Fill in the blanks in the table below. What are the inpatient service days for June 2 and 3?

Day	12:00 census A/C	Nb	adm A/C	b	trf in	total A/C	Nb	dis A/C	Nb dis	trf out	11:59 census A/C	Nb	a/d	serv days A/C	Nb
6/1	48	2	2	1	1	51	3	1	2	1	49	1	1	50	1
6/2	49	1	3	1	2	54	2	4	1	2	48	1	1		
6/3			1	1	1			3	0	1			0		

4. Would a newborn ever be considered an a/d?

5. At this point, you have inpatient service days for three successive days. The total of these data, excluding newborns, for June 1, 2, and 3 is 145 (50 + 49 + 46). What will you need to know and do to get the hospital total inpatient service days for the entire month of June?

Assignment No. 1

Assignment No. 1 consists of two worksheets for calculating a month's inpatient census and inpatient service days. If your findings do not match the data for the 31st, you have made an error in either your column additions or on one or more of the horizontal lines above the total. You must correct this error to ensure the validity of the monthly totals. If your column additions are correct, try a daily recap on each line until you find the error.

Assignment No. 1, Worksheet No. 1

<table>
<tr><td colspan="15">Monthly Compilation of Inpatient Census
and Inpatient Service Days
May 200_</td></tr>
<tr>
<td></td>
<td colspan="2">12:00
census</td>
<td>adm</td>
<td></td>
<td>trf</td>
<td colspan="2">total</td>
<td>dis</td>
<td>Nb</td>
<td>trf</td>
<td colspan="2">11:59
census</td>
<td></td>
<td colspan="2">serv
days</td>
</tr>
<tr>
<td>Day</td><td>A/C</td><td>Nb</td><td>A/C</td><td>b</td><td>in</td><td>A/C</td><td>Nb</td><td>A/C</td><td>dis</td><td>out</td><td>A/C</td><td>Nb</td><td>a/d</td><td>A/C</td><td>Nb</td>
</tr>
<tr><td>1</td><td>162</td><td>2</td><td>22</td><td>1</td><td>10</td><td>194</td><td>3</td><td>19</td><td>0</td><td>10</td><td>165</td><td>3</td><td>1</td><td>166</td><td>3</td></tr>
<tr><td>2</td><td>165</td><td>3</td><td>29</td><td>0</td><td>8</td><td></td><td></td><td>23</td><td>1</td><td>8</td><td></td><td></td><td></td><td></td><td></td></tr>
<tr><td>3</td><td></td><td></td><td>14</td><td>2</td><td>3</td><td></td><td></td><td>24</td><td>0</td><td>3</td><td></td><td></td><td>1</td><td></td><td></td></tr>
<tr><td>4</td><td></td><td></td><td>24</td><td>0</td><td>5</td><td></td><td></td><td>25</td><td>0</td><td>5</td><td></td><td></td><td></td><td></td><td></td></tr>
<tr><td>5</td><td></td><td></td><td>11</td><td>1</td><td>6</td><td></td><td></td><td>25</td><td>2</td><td>6</td><td></td><td></td><td></td><td></td><td></td></tr>
<tr><td>6</td><td></td><td></td><td>20</td><td>0</td><td>1</td><td></td><td></td><td>16</td><td>0</td><td>1</td><td></td><td></td><td></td><td></td><td></td></tr>
<tr><td>7</td><td></td><td></td><td>29</td><td>0</td><td>10</td><td></td><td></td><td>17</td><td>0</td><td>10</td><td></td><td></td><td></td><td></td><td></td></tr>
<tr><td>8</td><td></td><td></td><td>24</td><td>2</td><td>13</td><td></td><td></td><td>20</td><td>0</td><td>13</td><td></td><td></td><td>3</td><td></td><td></td></tr>
<tr><td>9</td><td></td><td></td><td>23</td><td>1</td><td>7</td><td></td><td></td><td>22</td><td>1</td><td>7</td><td></td><td></td><td>1</td><td></td><td></td></tr>
<tr><td>10</td><td></td><td></td><td>19</td><td>0</td><td>10</td><td></td><td></td><td>17</td><td>0</td><td>10</td><td></td><td></td><td></td><td></td><td></td></tr>
<tr><td>11</td><td></td><td></td><td>11</td><td>0</td><td>5</td><td></td><td></td><td>22</td><td>3</td><td>5</td><td></td><td></td><td>1</td><td></td><td></td></tr>
<tr><td>12</td><td></td><td></td><td>16</td><td>0</td><td>6</td><td></td><td></td><td>24</td><td>0</td><td>6</td><td></td><td></td><td></td><td></td><td></td></tr>
<tr><td>13</td><td></td><td></td><td>18</td><td>1</td><td>5</td><td></td><td></td><td>25</td><td>0</td><td>5</td><td></td><td></td><td></td><td></td><td></td></tr>
<tr><td>14</td><td></td><td></td><td>29</td><td>0</td><td>5</td><td></td><td></td><td>19</td><td>0</td><td>5</td><td></td><td></td><td></td><td></td><td></td></tr>
<tr><td>15</td><td></td><td></td><td>28</td><td>0</td><td>8</td><td></td><td></td><td>22</td><td>2</td><td>8</td><td></td><td></td><td>1</td><td></td><td></td></tr>
<tr><td>16</td><td></td><td></td><td>26</td><td>3</td><td>6</td><td></td><td></td><td>19</td><td>0</td><td>6</td><td></td><td></td><td></td><td></td><td></td></tr>
<tr><td>17</td><td></td><td></td><td>26</td><td>0</td><td>7</td><td></td><td></td><td>19</td><td>2</td><td>7</td><td></td><td></td><td></td><td></td><td></td></tr>
<tr><td>18</td><td></td><td></td><td>18</td><td>0</td><td>10</td><td></td><td></td><td>25</td><td>0</td><td>10</td><td></td><td></td><td></td><td></td><td></td></tr>
<tr><td>19</td><td></td><td></td><td>12</td><td>0</td><td>6</td><td></td><td></td><td>33</td><td>0</td><td>6</td><td></td><td></td><td></td><td></td><td></td></tr>
<tr><td>20</td><td></td><td></td><td>22</td><td>1</td><td>8</td><td></td><td></td><td>16</td><td>3</td><td>8</td><td></td><td></td><td>1</td><td></td><td></td></tr>
<tr><td>21</td><td></td><td></td><td>26</td><td>0</td><td>3</td><td></td><td></td><td>17</td><td>0</td><td>3</td><td></td><td></td><td>1</td><td></td><td></td></tr>
<tr><td>22</td><td></td><td></td><td>32</td><td>2</td><td>11</td><td></td><td></td><td>25</td><td>0</td><td>11</td><td></td><td></td><td>1</td><td></td><td></td></tr>
<tr><td>23</td><td></td><td></td><td>29</td><td>2</td><td>14</td><td></td><td></td><td>27</td><td>0</td><td>14</td><td></td><td></td><td></td><td></td><td></td></tr>
<tr><td>24</td><td></td><td></td><td>22</td><td>0</td><td>10</td><td></td><td></td><td>21</td><td>2</td><td>10</td><td></td><td></td><td></td><td></td><td></td></tr>
<tr><td>25</td><td></td><td></td><td>20</td><td>3</td><td>13</td><td></td><td></td><td>34</td><td>0</td><td>13</td><td></td><td></td><td></td><td></td><td></td></tr>
<tr><td>26</td><td></td><td></td><td>14</td><td>0</td><td>6</td><td></td><td></td><td>37</td><td>1</td><td>6</td><td></td><td></td><td>1</td><td></td><td></td></tr>
<tr><td>27</td><td></td><td></td><td>23</td><td>0</td><td>5</td><td></td><td></td><td>16</td><td>0</td><td>5</td><td></td><td></td><td></td><td></td><td></td></tr>
<tr><td>28</td><td></td><td></td><td>26</td><td>2</td><td>4</td><td></td><td></td><td>18</td><td>2</td><td>4</td><td></td><td></td><td></td><td></td><td></td></tr>
<tr><td>29</td><td></td><td></td><td>17</td><td>0</td><td>6</td><td></td><td></td><td>22</td><td>1</td><td>6</td><td></td><td></td><td>1</td><td></td><td></td></tr>
<tr><td>30</td><td></td><td></td><td>19</td><td>0</td><td>7</td><td></td><td></td><td>21</td><td>1</td><td>7</td><td></td><td></td><td></td><td></td><td></td></tr>
<tr><td>31</td><td>141</td><td>2</td><td>21</td><td>1</td><td>12</td><td>174</td><td>3</td><td>16</td><td>0</td><td>12</td><td>146</td><td>3</td><td>1</td><td>147</td><td>3</td></tr>
</table>

Assignment No. 1, Worksheet No. 2

Recap of Monthly Data for Adults and Children:

12:00 census A/C		162
adm A/C	+	_____
trf in	+	_____
total A/C	=	_____
dis A/C	−	_____
trf out	−	_____
11:59 census A/C	=	146

Recap of Monthly Data for Newborns:

12:00 census Nb		2
b	+	_____
total Nb	=	_____
Nb dis	−	_____
11:59 census Nb	=	3

serv days A/C (total inpatient service days excluding newborns) _____

serv days Nb (total newborn service days) _____

Total inpatient service days _____

Test on Computation of Census and Inpatient Service Days

Complete sections A through C.

Section A

1. Fill in the blanks in the chart below.

Day	12:00 census A/C	12:00 census Nb	adm A/C	b	trf in	total A/C	total Nb	dis A/C	Nb dis	trf out	11:59 census A/C	11:59 census Nb	a/d	serv days A/C	serv days Nb
6/1	250	18	20	4	2			25	3	2			1		
6/2			22	6	1			24	5	1			0		

2. If for the rest of the month there were 7,000 inpatient service days without newborns and 600 with newborns, how many total inpatient service days would there be for June?

3. Would leaving off the two transfer columns above make any changes in the census or inpatient service days?

Section B

1. Suppose 200 patients, including newborns, were in the hospital at midnight (11:59 P.M.) on August 31. During September, the following data are compiled:

   Admissions
      Adults and children   1,450
      Newborns   100
   Discharges (including deaths)
      Adults and children   1,400
      Newborns   95

   What would the inpatient census be at 11:59 P.M., September 30 (including newborns)?

2. Can you compute the inpatient service days with the information supplied in the previous question? Explain.

Section C

Unit A, a surgical unit, has reported the following data:

Day	12:00 census	adm	trf in	total	dis	trf out	11:59 census	a/d	serv days
6/1	50	6	1	59	9	1	49	1	50

Do these data look correct? Explain.

Average Daily Census

The *average daily census* is the average number of inpatients present each day for a given period of time. The *total inpatient service days* for any period (usually a month or a year) represents the inpatient service days for all the calendar days in that period. The formula for calculating average daily census is:

$$\frac{\textit{Total inpatient service days for a period (excluding newborns)}}{\textit{Total number of days in period}}$$

For question 2 in section A of the test on computation of census and inpatient service days, the answer was 7,489 inpatient service days for adults and children and 639 inpatient service days for newborns for the month of September. According to the formula, the average daily census, or average number of patients in the hospital each day of the month, is computed by dividing 7,489 by 30 (number of days in September). The result is 249.63, or, rounded to a whole number, 250. Because patient load can fluctuate, the administration is very interested in the hospital's average daily census. For example, many healthcare facilities in Florida experience a rise in average daily census during the winter months and a decrease during the summer months due to seasonal visitors. The average daily census is a measure of use and a reference for anticipated revenues.

As mentioned earlier, adults and children are calculated separately from newborns unless otherwise directed by the hospital's administration. Newborn census data tend to distort statistics related to resource use. For example, it costs less to maintain a newborn nursery than it does to staff other PCUs. If the average daily census is consistently low over a specified period, it may be appropriate to close PCUs to reduce expenses. In this example, the average daily newborn census is calculated by dividing 639 by 30. The result is 21.3, or 21.

Whether to round to a whole number is the individual hospital's decision. What is important is that the hospital act consistently. There is a difference between working with data representing people (because you cannot have a portion of a person) and working with percentages that represent numbers. (Rounding numbers is discussed in chapter 1.)

Another example of average daily census is that of a 100-bed hospital that compiles 2,480 inpatient service days for July. To compute the average daily census for July, divide 2,480 by 31 (number of days in July). The average daily census is 80.

Average Daily Newborn Census

When administrators and physicians ask for the average daily census, they may not always indicate to exclude newborns. Clarify the information by asking if newborns should be included or excluded from your computations. The formula for calculating the average daily census for newborns follows the same pattern as the formula for calculating the average daily census of adults and children:

$$\frac{\textit{Total newborn inpatient service days for a period}}{\textit{Total number of days in the period}}$$

For example, a hospital with 30 bassinets had 800 newborn inpatient service days during June. Divide the total number of newborn inpatient service days (800) by the number of days in the period (30 days in June) to obtain the average daily newborn census (26.6666, or 27).

Average Daily Census for a Care Unit

It is often helpful for the hospital's administration to know the average use of a specific medical care unit (for example, to know whether additional beds are needed for the ICU). Statistics do not make decisions, but they are the basis for decision making. The formula for calculating the average daily census for a care unit is:

$$\frac{\textit{Total inpatient service days for the unit for the period}}{\textit{Total number of days in the period}}$$

Exercise 2.6

1. XYZ hospital has 210 beds and 30 newborn bassinets. Total inpatient service days for February, in a nonleap year, were 5,620 for adults and children and 743 for newborns. What is the average daily census (rounded to a whole number)?

2. A 100-bed, 10-bassinet hospital has 2,641 inpatient service days for adults and children and 232 newborn service days during June. What is the average daily census (excluding newborns)?

3. Compute the average daily newborn census for a 100-bed, 10-bassinet hospital with 2,641 inpatient service days for adults and children and 232 inpatient service days for newborns during June. Round your answer to a whole number.

4. If you need to calculate the average daily census of the ICU, where can you obtain the ICU's inpatient service days?

5. Using the following statistics from an actual report generated monthly by the nursing administration of an acute care facility, calculate the current month's (June) average daily census for each nursing unit and the totals to validate this report. Note that this facility's policy is not to round to a whole number but, instead, to carry the average daily census to the hundredth.

Memorial Hospital
Inpatient Statistical Report
Average Daily Census by Nursing Unit
10/01/99 thru 6/30/00

		Month Inpt Serv days	Current Month	This month last year	Current FY to date	Previous FY to date
A.	Obstetrical	545	18.16	26.40	17.64	26.06
B.	Pediatric	454	15.13	17.36	16.07	17.85
C.	Med/Surg	5023	167.43	161.33	200.90	196.06
D.	Med ICU	271	9.03	6.56	12.20	12.15
E.	Surg ICU	250	8.33	8.33	10.86	10.75
F.	Med Prog Care	593	19.76	29.06	24.76	40.21
G.	Surg Prog Care	569	18.96	16.63	22.85	21.90
H.	Open Heart ICU	164	5.46	2.70	5.77	4.95
	Total Adult & Children	**7869**	**262.30**	**268.40**	**311.10**	**329.96**
I.	Normal Nb	378	12.60	15.86	13.51	14.87
J.	Prog Care Nurse	126	4.20	.00	7.12	3.05
K.	Neonatal ICU	392	13.06	15.50	9.85	12.89
	Total Nursery	**896**	**29.86**	**31.36**	**30.49**	**30.82**

Test on Average Daily Census

Complete sections A and B.

Section A

In 1995, a hospital had 160 beds for adults and children from January 1 through June 30. On July 1, the hospital increased its beds to 200 and the number remained at 200 through December 31. During the first six months, 26,510 patient days of service were provided to the hospital's adults and children. During the last six months, 33,910 days of service were provided. Answer the following questions and round the answers to whole numbers:

1. What was the average daily census for the entire year?

    a.   146
    b.   153
    c.   166
    d.   184

2. What was the average daily census for the first six months?

    a.   145
    b.   146
    c.   147
    d.   148

3. The same hospital provided 6,590 newborn days of service in its 20-bassinet nursery during the year. What was the average daily newborn census?

    a.   15
    b.   16
    c.   17
    d.   18

Section B

A hospital medical unit has 50 beds. During August, the unit provided 1,420 days of service.

What was the average daily census for the medical unit in August?

a.   28
b.   45
c.   46
d.   47

Chapter 3
Bed Occupancy Ratio

Objectives

At the conclusion of this chapter, you should be able to:

- Define and differentiate among the terms *bed count, newborn bed count, bed count days,* and *newborn bed count days*

- Compute the bed occupancy ratio for any period given the data representing bed count and inpatient service days

- Compute the bassinet occupancy ratio for any period given bassinet count and newborn inpatient service days

Bed Count

Typically, a healthcare facility is licensed by the state to operate with a specific number of beds. If a new facility wants to open its doors for patient care, it must apply for a certificate of need (CON) to prove that patient care beds are needed in the region. If granted a CON by the state, the facility then is licensed for a specific number of beds and is responsible for reporting its bed count.

A *bed count* is the number of available facility inpatient beds, both occupied and vacant, on any given day. In a hospital, the bed count includes those beds set up for normal use, whether or not they are occupied. A bed count may be reported for the entire hospital or for any of its units. Normally, when counting inpatient beds, only those in space designed for such accommodations and set up, staffed, equipped, and in all respects ready for the care of patients are counted. This is an important consideration because regulatory agency surveyors often verify bed count and location against licensed beds and appropriate staffing levels.

The types of beds to be excluded from the bed count are those in treatment areas such as examining rooms, emergency services, physical therapy, labor rooms, and recovery rooms. Newborn beds, called bassinets, are computed separately from the bed count. The *newborn bassinet count* is the number of available hospital newborn bassinets, both occupied and vacant, on any given day.

The bed count may be used in various reports. For example, in 1993, a membership survey was sent to AHIMA members. The number of surveys returned was 18,834. One of the items included in the survey was facility bed size (count). Table 3.1 shows the responses.

From the responses, it can be determined that 19.4 percent of the respondents worked in small facilities (1–99 beds); 49.4 percent (31.4 + 18.0) worked in mid-sized facilities (100–499); 13.2 percent (11.5 + 1.7) worked in large facilities; and 17.9 percent worked in non-acute care facilities or nontraditional settings.

In a hospital, the number of available beds in a facility or a unit may remain constant for long periods of time. At times, however, the number can and does change. For example, a significant number of beds may be unavailable for use during a major remodeling or renovation. Therefore, it is always wise to do a bed count.

The term *bed complement* is an alternate term for bed count. The term *bed capacity* also has been used synonymously with bed count and bed complement, but its use has led to some confusion. Bed capacity also can denote the number of beds that a facility has been designed and constructed to contain, rather than the actual number of beds set up and staffed for use. To avoid confusion, it is preferable to use the term *bed count*.

Table 3.1.	AHIMA Membership Survey, 1993	
	Facility Bed Size	**% of Respondents**
	1–99	19.4%
	100–299	31.4%
	300–499	18.0%
	500–999	11.5%
	> 1,000	1.7%
	Not applicable	17.9%

Two areas may cause some controversy in bed count. One area concerns labor room beds because the patient may be admitted directly to a labor bed instead of to a postpartum bed where she may spend the majority of her hospital stay. Generally, however, labor room beds are not included in the bed count.

The second area of controversy concerns emergency department (ED) beds. Normally, ED beds are considered outpatient beds. The patient is not admitted to the hospital formally until he or she leaves. In some instances, however, the hospital provides an observation bed in the ED. If observation beds meet the qualifications of being set up, equipped, and staffed for inpatient use, they may be counted, depending on what the particular facility has decided as well as on state-licensing compliance.

A patient under observation (a so-called observation patient) needs to be monitored, evaluated, and assessed for admission to inpatient status or discharged for care to another setting. He or she can occupy a special bed set aside for this purpose or a bed in any unit of a hospital (that is, the ED, a medical unit, or obstetrics). Hospitals need terms to describe and classify outpatients who occupy hospital beds and information systems to track these patients.

Exercise 3.1

In the event of a disaster, extra beds are available that may be set up to meet the immediate needs of the disaster situation. Are these beds part of the bed count?

Bed Count Days

A *bed count day* is a unit of measure denoting the presence of one inpatient bed (either occupied or vacant) set up and staffed for use in one 24-hour period. The term *total bed count days* refers to the sum of inpatient bed count days for each of the days in the period under consideration. Bed count days also may be referred to as the maximum number of patient days or potential days because they represent a statistical probability of every bed being occupied every day.

If every hospital bed were filled each day for a certain period (for example, a month), the occupancy rate would be 100 percent. This is because the bed was occupied the maximum number of times it could have been occupied. It is important to note that a rate is the number of times something occurred compared to the number of times something could have occurred. (See chapter 2.) The number of times it actually occurred is expressed in terms of inpatient service days. The number of times it could have occurred is expressed in terms of bed count days (bed count multiplied by the number of calendar days).

Bed Occupancy Ratio

The *bed occupancy ratio* is the proportion of beds occupied, defined as the ratio of inpatient service days to bed count days in the period under consideration. The inpatient census represents the actual occupancy (number of occurrences) and the bed count represents the possibility for occupancy (number of times it could have occurred or the maximum possible). The formula for determining bed occupancy ratio is:

$$\frac{\text{Total inpatient service days in a period} \times 100}{\text{Total bed count days in the period (Bed count} \times \text{Number of days in the period)}}$$

Synonymous terms for bed occupancy ratio are *percent occupancy, occupancy percent, percentage of occupancy,* and *occupancy ratio.* The ratio is usually expressed as a percent and can be computed at a specified time (for example, 12 A.M.), for any specified day, or as a daily average in any period of time.

For example, on June 1, 170 inpatient service days were provided in a 200-bed hospital. Making the appropriate substitutions in the previously stated formula, the bed occupancy ratio is calculated as follows:

$$\frac{(170 \times 100)}{200} = \frac{17,000}{200} = 85\%$$

The bed occupancy ratio for June 1 is 85 percent.

You might prefer to compute a decimal fraction and then multiply by 100. Or convert to a percentage by moving the decimal point two places to the right as:

$$\frac{17,000}{200} = .85 = 85\%$$

Here is another example of bed occupancy ratio for the period of a month. In December, 1,400 inpatient service days were provided at a hospital that is licensed for 50 beds. Taking into account that December has 31 days, the bed occupancy ratio is calculated as follows:

$$\frac{(1,400 \times 100)}{(50 \times 31)} = \frac{140,000}{1,550} = 90.3\%$$

The bed occupancy ratio for December is 90.3 percent.

Change in Bed Count

Occasionally, a hospital changes its bed count during a period. This expansion or reduction is a permanent change and is not designed to meet an emergency situation. For example, a hospital changes its official bed count from 50 to 75 on January 15 and goes on to provide a total of 1,700 inpatient service days for the entire month. How is the maximum number of bed count days determined for the month of January? Multiply 50 beds by the first 14 days of the month and 75 beds by the 17 remaining days of the month, and then add the products.

$$14 \times 50 = 700$$

$$17 \times 75 = 1{,}275$$

$$700 + 1{,}275 = 1{,}975$$

The maximum number of bed count days for January is 1,975. Now compute the bed occupancy ratio. The resulting calculation is:

$$\frac{(1{,}700 \times 100)}{1{,}975} = \frac{170{,}000}{1{,}975} = 86.07 = 86.1\%$$

The bed occupancy ratio for January is 86.1 percent.

This procedure provides the most accurate result. Compare the previous computation with what would have happened if 50 beds had been used for the entire month:

$$\frac{(1{,}700 \times 100)}{(50 \times 31)} = \frac{170{,}000}{1{,}550} = 109.67 = 109.7\%$$

If 75 beds had been used for the entire month, the calculation would be:

$$\frac{(1{,}700 \times 100)}{(75 \times 31)} = \frac{170{,}000}{2{,}325} = 73.11 = 73.1\%$$

Obviously, there is a significant difference in the results (86.1, 109.7, and 73.1 percent). This example illustrates how easy it can be to present an inaccurate statistical picture. Many administrative decisions are made on the basis of statistical presentations. The HIM practitioner has an important responsibility in providing accurate statistics as well as validating computerized statistics.

Newborn Bassinet Occupancy Ratio

Normally, newborn occupancy ratios are computed separately. If every bassinet were full every day in the period, the hospital would have the maximum potential bassinet occupancy. The formula for determining newborn bassinet occupancy is:

$$\frac{\textit{Total newborn inpatient service days for a period} \times 100}{\textit{Total newborn bassinet count} \times \textit{Number of days in the period}}$$

For example, during March, a hospital with a bassinet count of 30 provided 810 newborn inpatient service days of care. According to the formula, the newborn bassinet occupancy ratio for March is:

$$\frac{(810 \times 100)}{(30 \times 31)} = \frac{81{,}000}{930} = 87.09\% = 87.1\%$$

Exercise 3.2

1. On December 10, 55 inpatient service days were given to patients in a hospital with a bed count of 75. What was the bed occupancy ratio (percent of occupancy) for December 10?

2. A 100-bed hospital had 2,590 inpatient service days in February (during a non-leap year). The bed occupancy ratio is 9.25 percent. True or false?

3. A 250-bed hospital determined that its bed occupancy ratio was not high enough to meet its debts. On July 17, an administrative decision was made to close a patient care unit, which decreased the official bed count to 200. During July, 5,650 inpatient service days were provided. What was the bed occupancy ratio for July?

4. A hospital provided 200 newborn inpatient service days in its 20-bassinet nursery in November. The bassinet occupancy ratio for this hospital is 33.3 percent. True or false?

5. Write down the formula for computing a PCU's percentage of occupancy (bed occupancy ratio).

Bed Turnover Rate

The *bed turnover rate* is defined as the number of times a bed, on average, changes occupants during a given period of time. It is another measure of hospital utilization. The bed turnover rate demonstrates the net effect of changes in occupancy rate and length of stay. (LOS is discussed in chapter 4.)

Following are two formulas for determining bed turnover rate. The direct formula is:

$$\frac{Number\ of\ discharges\ (including\ deaths)\ for\ a\ period}{Average\ bed\ count\ during\ the\ period}$$

The indirect formula is:

$$\frac{Occupancy\ rate \times Number\ of\ days\ in\ a\ period}{Average\ length\ of\ stay}$$

There is no universal agreement on the most accurate formula. However, the two formulas, although computed differently, yield basically the same results. The following example displays both formulas and yields basically the same turnover rate for a short-stay hospital.

A 200-bed hospital supplied the following information for the year 1999: patients discharged and died, 6,500; average length of stay, 9 days; and bed occupancy rate, 80 percent.

$$\text{Direct formula: } \frac{6,500}{200} = 32.5$$

$$\text{Indirect formula: } \frac{(.8 \times 365)}{9} = \frac{292}{9} = 32.4$$

Note that in the indirect formula the bed occupancy rate must be changed to a decimal. This example shows that during 1999, each of the hospital's 200 beds changed occupants about 32.5 times.

While there is no universal agreement on the most accurate formula, administrators of short-stay hospitals are becoming increasingly interested in bed turnover rates as a measure of hospital utilization, especially when related as a rate to occupancy and length of stay. When occupancy goes up and length of stay goes down, or vice versa, the bed turnover rate makes it easier to see the net effect of these changes. Turnover rates can be used in comparing one facility with another or in comparing utilization rates for different time periods or for different units of the same facility. For example, the occupancy rate for one hospital can be essentially the same in two time periods, but the turnover rate may be lower because of a longer length of stay in one time period. In other words, bed turnover rate can be a measure of intensity of utilization.

Exercise 3.3

Using the statistics in the following actual report generated for a medical center, calculate the occupancy rates to validate the report.

ABC Medical Center
April 1999

	Patient days	Bed count	Occupancy
Med/Surg	2883	143	67.2%
Critical care	277	13	70.8%
Stepdown	225	13	57.7%
Rehab	373	25	49.6%
OB	328	30	36.3%
Psychiatry	412	28	48.9%
Neonatal ICU	281	12	78.3%
Pediatrics	125	10	42.0%
Total	**4904**	**274**	**59.6%**
Nursery	138	16	28.8%

Test on Bed Occupancy Ratio

Complete sections A and B.

Section A

A hospital compiled the following statistics for 1998:

Inpatient service days:		**Newborn service days:**	11,500
January–June	26,510	**Newborn bassinet count:**	40
July–December	33,910		
(December 31 only	185)		

Bed count:
January–June	160
July–December	200

Select the correct answer to each of the following questions, rounding off to the first position after the decimal.

1. The inpatient bed occupancy ratio (without newborns) for 1998 was:

   a. 91.8%
   b. 91.9%
   c. 92.0%
   d. 92.1%

2. The newborn bassinet occupancy ratio for 1998 was:

   a. 78.7%
   b. 78.8%
   c. 78.9%
   d. 79.0%

3. The bed occupancy ratio for December 31 was:

   a. 77.1%
   b. 92.5%
   c. 115.6%
   d. 120.1%

Section B

The following table is an actual report of the first quarter of 1999 (January–March) from a 450-bed medical center.

Medical Center
Patient Days and Discharges by Sponsor
January–March 1999

Sponsor	Patient Days	Number of Patients Discharged
Contracts	3,749	565
Medicare	7,154	891
Medicaid	11,156	1,782
County	4,615	769
Private Pay	2,397	358
Nonsponsor	838	166
Total	**29,909**	**4,531**

1. Calculate the occupancy rate (percentage of occupancy) for:

   a. total
   b. Medicare
   c. private pay

2. Calculate the bed turnover rate using the direct formula for:

    a. total

    b. Medicare

    c. private pay

Assignment No. 2

Using data from the assignment in chapter 2, compute the following averages and ratios. The hospital has an inpatient bed count of 210 and a bassinet count of 10. Round your answers to one place beyond the decimal. Remember that newborns are considered separately.

1. Average daily census

2. Average daily newborn census

3. Bed occupancy ratio for the month

4. Bassinet occupancy ratio for the month

5. Bed occupancy ratio for May 25

Chapter 4
Length of Stay Data

Objectives

At the conclusion of this chapter, you should be able to:

- Compute average length of stay using the formulas provided
- Compute the average length of stay for newborns using the formula provided
- Compute the length of stay for one patient based on data provided
- Compute the total length of stay for a group of discharged patients
- Determine the median length of stay for small groups of patients
- Describe the conditions under which the median is the preferred measure of central tendency when presenting average length of stay

Length of Stay

Length of stay (LOS) is the number of calendar days a patient stays in the hospital, from admission to discharge. The healthcare facility uses LOS data in utilization management. Utilization management evaluates the facility's efficiency in providing necessary services in the most cost-effective manner, while also evaluating the level of care required. Its goal is to eliminate over- and underutilization of services. Part of the utilization management process involves reviewing LOS for continued medical necessity. For example, is it more appropriate to continue to treat the patient in an acute care facility or to transfer the patient to a subacute or rehabilitation facility?

LOS data also are used in financial reports, for example, to compare patients within the same diagnosis-related group (DRG). A particular DRG average length of stay (ALOS) can be compared to the healthcare facility's DRG ALOS to note whether there are too many extreme values (outliers). LOS data for patients with the same diagnosis or procedure treated by various physicians are compared to evaluate any extremes.

Discharge Days

In chapter 2, you worked with service days, which are compiled on a continuing basis while the patient is hospitalized. In this chapter, you will work with discharge days, which are days compiled on the patient after he or she has been discharged from the hospital. Synonymous terms for length of stay include *days of stay, inpatient days of stay, duration of inpatient hospitalization,* and *discharge days.*

The LOS for one patient is determined by subtracting the date of admission from the date of discharge when the patient is admitted and discharged within the same month. The day of admission is counted in computing the number of discharge days or LOS, but the day of discharge is not. When the patient's stay extends beyond one or more months, days must be added to calculate the LOS. The LOS is one day if the patient is admitted and discharged on the same day.

Following is an example of how to calculate LOS for the following discharged patients:

Date Admitted	Date Discharged	Length of Stay
6/25	6/25	1 day
6/25	6/26	1 day
6/25	6/30	5 days
6/25	7/4	9 days (6 days in June + 3 days in July)
6/25	8/4	40 days (6 days in June + 31 days in July + 3 days in August)

Exercise 4.1

Calculate the LOS for the following discharged patients:

Date Admitted	Date Discharged	Length of Stay
8/1	8/17	
8/27	9/1	
8/15	8/15	
8/3	8/4	
12/1/98	2/8/99	

Total Length of Stay

The *total length of stay* (for all inpatients) is the sum of the days' stay of any group of inpatients discharged during a specified period of time. Total length of stay also may be referred to as *discharge days*. Although the total length of stay and inpatient service days may approximate each other over a long period of time, they are not interchangeable. The reason for this is that inpatient service days are counted concurrently and discharge days are counted after discharge.

For example, a patient hospitalized for a period beyond an entire year and into a second year (for example, a rehabilitation patient) would be credited with 365 inpatient service days at the end of the first year, but no discharge days. When the patient is discharged from the hospital in the second year, all of the discharge days from admission to discharge are counted at that time, increasing the discharge days for the second year by at least 365.

If the patient stays in the hospital for two or more years (as happens in longer-term institutions), all of the 730+ days are assigned to one year in calculating duration of inpatient hospitalization. These types of patients increase the number of discharge days for any year, making the total number much larger than inpatient service days for the same period.

Why calculate both inpatient days of service (census days) and total length of stay (discharge days)? Each is meaningful in its own right. Inpatient service days are useful in the analysis of current utilization of hospital facilities related to the entire hospital, a clinical unit, or a service department. They are used to compute various daily averages and occupancy ratios. The total length of stay can be used to analyze LOS for groups of discharged patients with similar characteristics such as age, disease, treatment, clinical service, or day of week admitted.

Exercise 4.2

Using the table below, first calculate the total length of stay (discharge days) for the 10 patients listed and then calculate the total length of stay for:

A. Medical patients
B. Surgical patients
C. Obstetrical patients
D. Patients younger than 16 years old
E. Patients 16–30 years old
F. Patients 31–64 years old
G. Patients 65 years old or older

Patients Discharged 12/1/99

Name	Age	Clinical Service	Length of Stay
Jones	52	Medical	15
Smith	5	Surgical	1
Shultz	69	Medical	37
Valdez	22	Obstetrical	1
Johnson	10	Surgical	7
O'Brien	80	Surgical	8
Chu	26	Obstetrical	2
Martini	49	Medical	42
Lewandowski	35	Surgical	11
MacDuff	18	Obstetrical	3

Average Length of Stay

Average length of stay (ALOS) is the average number of days that inpatients discharged during the period under consideration stayed in the hospital. The formula for calculating ALOS is:

$$\frac{Total\ length\ of\ stay\ (discharge\ days)}{Total\ discharges\ (including\ deaths)}$$

For example, the American Hospital Association (AHA) reported that the ALOS for inpatients declined to an all-time low of 6.1 days in 1997, with the overall inpatient days dropping to 12.9 percent. Comparatively, the ALOS for patients under age 65 was 4.9 days in 1994, a reduction of 0.3 days from 1993. Several trends in healthcare have contributed to this reduction in ALOS, including managed care, home healthcare, skilled nursing units in hospitals, and an increase in outpatient visits. Synonymous terms for average length of stay include *average duration of hospitalization* and *average stay.*

The formula above does not include the ALOS for newborns. Most hospitals calculate the ALOS for newborns separately because newborns generally stay the same length of time as their mothers. In addition, when compared to many other classifications of patients, newborn stays are relatively short. Therefore, inclusion of both mothers and newborns would distort the total ALOS.

The ALOS for the 10 patients listed in exercise 4.2 is 12.7 or 13 days ($^{127}/_{10}$). Based on the information in the table, the ALOS for medical patients is 31 days ($^{94}/_{3}$), and the ALOS for patients under the age of 16 is 4 days ($^{8}/_{2}$).

Options for Avoiding Distortions

As discussed previously, a long-stay patient's discharge days are allocated to the period in which he or she is discharged. Sometimes this can give a distorted average, especially on a monthly (rather than annual) basis. For example, in March, a hospital discharged 130 patients with a total length of stay of 1,267. The LOS for one of the patients was 365 days. The ALOS for all 130 patients was 9.7 or 10 days ($^{1,267}/_{130} = 9.74$). If the stay of the one patient is removed from the total length of stay, the ALOS becomes 6.99 or 7 days (1,267 − 365 = 902; $^{902}/_{129} = 6.99$). Should one patient or a few patients in a population affect the average to this degree? Is the statistical computation meaningful for decision-making purposes? In this situation, the hospital has two options:

- *Option 1:* A notation can be made on the report that either the ALOS of 10 includes one patient who stayed a year or the ALOS of 7 excludes one patient who stayed a year. Both calculations can be made. Appropriate notes should be attached to the report to indicate the difference.

- *Option 2:* The computation using the median rather than the mean can be used. As discussed in chapter 1, the *median* is the midpoint of a series (that is, the point above which and below which 50 percent of the numbers lie). For the series, ordered numbers are arranged in numerical order from highest to lowest, or vice versa.

Median Used in Average Length of Stay

Looking at exercise 4.2, the list in the table includes the LOS of 10 discharged patients. These numbers placed in order from high to low are: 42, 37, 15, 11, 8, 7, 3, 2, 1, 1. The midpoint falls halfway between 7 and 8, or 7.5. Note that, regardless of value, 50 percent of the total numbers fall above this point and 50 percent fall below. The median provides a more revealing representation of the ALOS when one or a few long-stay patients would otherwise distort the arithmetic mean. The median is not sensitive to outliers as is the mean. Obviously, manual computation of the median is much more time-consuming than computation of the mean. Moreover, it would be impractical with a large number of discharged patients. Therefore, if the statistical computation is manual, it would be better to use option 1 above. However, if the statistical computation is computerized, it would be better to use option 2.

According to the table in exercise 4.2, medical patients stayed 42, 37, and 15 days for a total of 94 days. Using the formula, the ALOS for medical patients is 31.3 ($^{94}/_3$). The median or midpoint is 37. Obviously, the mean, or average, according to the formula is a better method to use here because there are no unusually long or short stays. However, there is an unusually long stay in the group aged 31 to 64.

Exercise 4.3

1. In January, a hospital reported 794 discharge days for adults and children and 84 discharge days for newborns. During the month, 142 adults and children and 28 newborns were discharged. What was the ALOS (rounded to one decimal place) for the month of January?

2. Using the table in exercise 4.2, compute the ALOS and the median for the group of patients between ages 31 and 64. The ALOS is 22.7 days, and the median is 15. True or false?

3. Following is an actual report from Community Hospital for April 1999. Verify the calculations for ALOS and then rearrange the data into a more readable report.

Community Hospital
April, 1999

Discharges:

Med-surg/critical care and stepdown	670
Rehab	24
OB	157
Psychiatry	67
Neonatal ICU	11
Pediatrics	24
Total	**953**

Discharge days:

Med-surg/critical care and stepdown	3,390
Rehab	372
OB	329
Psychiatry	409
Neonatal ICU	280
Pediatrics	125
Total	**4,905**

Length of stay:

Med-surg/critical care and stepdown	5.1
Rehab	15.5
OB	2.1
Psychiatry	6.1
Neonatal ICU	25.5
Pediatrics	5.2
Total	**5.1**

Average Newborn Length of Stay

As stated earlier, newborn LOS is usually calculated separately. The discussion concerning a long stay affecting an ALOS also applies to newborns. The formula for calculating average newborn length of stay is:

$$\frac{Total\ newborn\ discharge\ days}{Total\ newborn\ discharges\ (including\ deaths)}$$

Exercise 4.4

Using the following data for a hospital during the month of February, what is the ALOS for newborns?

Newborn service days	510
Newborn discharge days	560
Newborn discharges	140
Births	135

Leave of Absence Days

Another data element that is significant in some hospitals is the number of leave of absence days. A *leave of absence* is the physician-authorized absence of an inpatient from a hospital or other facility for a specified period of time occurring after admission and prior to discharge. A leave of absence day is determined when the patient is not present at the census-taking hour.

Leave of absence data are important for administrative purposes as well as for the analysis of the services provided and care patterns. Days on leave of absence usually are excluded or tabulated separately when computing bed occupancy, calculating inpatient service days, or preparing inpatient census. Normally, they are included when considering discharge days and computing ALOS. Sometimes a hospital elects to discharge and then readmit the patient rather than grant a leave of absence.

Test on Length of Stay

Last year, a hospital compiled the following statistics:

Inpatient discharges

Total adult and children	10,810
Total newborn	1,601
Obstetrical	1,932
Medical	6,050
Surgical	2,828

Inpatient service days

Adult and children	60,420
Newborn	4,623

Discharge days

Total adult and children	73,104
Total newborn	4,808
Obstetrical	4,896
Medical	36,500
Surgical	31,708

Births 1,615

Section A

Using the statistics given, determine the following calculations.

1. The ALOS is:

    a. 5.6 days
    b. 5.8 days
    c. 6.3 days
    d. 6.8 days

2. The ALOS for surgical patients is 11.2 days.

    a. True
    b. False

3. The calculation for newborn ALOS is:

    a. $\dfrac{4,623}{1,615}$

    b. $\dfrac{4,808}{1,615}$

    c. $\dfrac{4,623}{1,601}$

    d. $\dfrac{4,808}{1,601}$

Section B

1. Determine the LOS for each of the following patients:

	Admitted	Discharged
a.	12/1/99	12/12/99
b.	12/12/99	12/13/99
c.	12/13/99	1/4/2000
d.	1/4/2000	1/4/2000
e.	12/13/99	1/9/2001

2. What is the total length of stay for this group of patients?

Section C

Under what circumstances is the median preferred over the mean in computing ALOS?

Section D

Calculate the ALOS for the following Medicare patients:

Patients	Medicare Discharge Days	Medicare Discharges
Acute	950	149
Rehabilitation	242	15
Skilled Nursing Facility	315	19

Chapter 5
Obstetrical and Perinatal Rates

Objectives

At the conclusion of this chapter, you should be able to:

- Define and differentiate among neonatal deaths, postneonatal deaths, and infant deaths
- Compute infant mortality rates and fetal death (stillborn) rates
- Compute maternal death rates
- Compute cesarean section rates

Infant Mortality Rate

Statistical tabulations for vital events related to pregnancy and newborns can provide valuable information on reproductive health. They also can provide data on national and international trends. Many of these rates are not calculated routinely by hospitals because infant and maternal deaths occur infrequently.

Table 5.1 lists infant mortality rates reported by the United Nations *Demographic Yearbook* for 1977, 1992, and 1995.

Table 5.1. **Infant Mortality Rates, United Nations *Demographic Yearbook***

Infant Mortality Rate—Deaths per 1,000 Births

Country	1977	1992	1995
Australia	14.3	9	6
Canada	15.0	7	6
Denmark	10.4	8	7
Finland	10.5	6	5
France	15.5	8	7
Japan	10.1	5	4
Norway	11.1	8	5
Sweden	8.1	6	5
UK	14.3	9	6
US	15.2	10	7

The following definitions were recommended in an issue of *Public Health Reports* (USPHS 1988). The terminology for reporting reproductive health statistics in the United States was approved by the American College of Obstetricians and Gynecologists in 1985 and was developed to promote uniform collection and interpretation of reproductive health statistics.

- *Neonatal death:* This term refers to the death of a liveborn infant within the period of 27 days, 23 hours, and 59 minutes from the moment of birth.

- *Postneonatal death:* This term refers to the death of a liveborn infant from 28 days of birth to the end of the first year of life (through 364 days, 23 hours, 59 minutes from the moment of birth).

- *Infant death:* This term refers to the death of a liveborn infant at any time from the moment of birth to the end of the first year of life (through 364 days, 23 hours, 59 minutes from the moment of birth).

Following is the formula for calculating the neonatal mortality rate:

$$\frac{\textit{Total number of newborn deaths for a period} \times 100}{\textit{Total number of newborn infant discharges (including deaths) for the period}}$$

When computing death rates, carry out the answer to at least two decimal places and do not round to a whole number. This is important because death rates are usually very small. When healthcare facilities report discharges, they typically include deaths in the discharge figures because a death is a type of a discharge. Or, as one student put it, "Death is the ultimate discharge." If a hospital had 2,000 newborn discharges for a year and one newborn death, its neonatal mortality rate would be calculated as:

$$\frac{(1 \times 100)}{2,000} = 0.05\%$$

Researchers frequently use birth certificate data for public health and policy studies. Similar vital statistics formulas are used in the United States. Following is a listing of vital statistics formulas:

Neonatal Mortality Rate Formula:

$$\frac{\textit{Number of neonatal deaths during a period} \times 1,000}{\textit{Number of live births during the period}}$$

Postneonatal Mortality Rate Formula:

$$\frac{\textit{Number of postneonatal deaths during a period} \times 1,000}{\textit{Number of live births during the period}}$$

Infant Mortality Rate Formula:

$$\frac{\textit{Number of infant deaths (neonatal and postneonatal)} \ \textit{during a period} \times 1,000}{\textit{Number of live births during the period}}$$

Using the same data cited previously (births 3,856; newborn deaths, 3; and newborn discharges, 3,850), the vital statistics neonatal mortality rate is calculated as follows:

$$\frac{(3 \times 1,000)}{3,856} = \frac{3,000}{3.856} = 0.7780 = 0.8 \ \textit{per} \ 1,000$$

Table 5.2 shows an actual report generated by a hospital for its medical staff perinatal committee. The hospital uses the vital statistics formula for neonatal mortality rate for the calculations.

Exercise 5.1

A hospital reports the following annual statistics: births, 3,856; newborn deaths, 3; and newborn discharges, 3,850. What is the hospital's neonatal mortality rate?

Table 5.2. Report for Medical Staff Perinatal Committee, 1988–1994

Memorial Health System
Perinatal Committee

Birth-Weight
Specific Mortality
(Deaths/1000 Live Births)

Calendar

Weight	Year 1988	Year 1989	Year 1990	Year 1991	Year 1992	Year 1993	Year 1994
<500 GMS	222.2	916.6	900.0	875.0	800.0	1000.0	700.0
500–749	750.0	857.1	444.4	666.6	428.6	500.0	571.4
750–999	555.6	400.0	71.4	133.3	90.9	222.2	0.0
1000–1499	58.8	0.0	0.0	0.0	41.7	111.1	76.9
1500–1999	6.7	39.2	20.0	20.4	0.0	0.0	0.0
2000–2499	4.7	5.9	0.0	10.2	0.0	0.0	21.7
2500–2999	2.6	0.0	0.0	0.0	2.0	1.9	1.8
3000+	0.3	0.4	0.4	0.3	0.8	0.0	0.0
Total Births	**4405**	**3615**	**3794**	**3537**	**3243**	**3070**	**3005**

Fetal Death Rate

A *hospital fetal death* is defined as a death prior to the complete expulsion or extraction from the mother (in a hospital facility) of a product of human conception (fetus and placenta) regardless of the duration of pregnancy. The death is indicated by the fact that after such expulsion or extraction, the fetus does not breathe or show any other evidence of life such as beating of the heart, pulsation of the umbilical cord, or definite movement of voluntary muscles. Typically, hospitals are required to report fetal deaths to a state agency. However, the reporting of fetal deaths varies according to individual state laws, statutes, and regulations. The formula for calculating fetal death rate is:

$$\frac{\text{Total number of intermediate and/or late fetal deaths for a period} \times 100}{\text{Total number of live births} + \text{Intermediate and late fetal deaths for the period}}$$

Because fetal deaths are not considered patient deaths, they are not included in any calculation of deaths but, rather, are calculated separately. Determination of whether to include fetal death data in a specific hospital's statistics requires an investigation of the facility's needs by hospital administration, medical staff, and reporting agencies. Fetal deaths may be classified as:

- *Early death:* Fewer than 20 weeks of gestation and a weight of 500 grams or less

- *Intermediate death:* Twenty completed weeks of gestation (but less than 28 weeks) and a weight of between 501 and 1,000 grams

- *Late death:* Twenty-eight completed weeks of gestation and a weight of more than 1,001 grams

Both intermediate and late fetal deaths constitute what is commonly termed a *still-birth*. The *ICD-9-CM* coding system contains definitions for *early fetal death* and *late fetal death* for classification purposes that differ from the above definitions.

For example, during June, a hospital had 100 live births, one intermediate fetal death, and three late fetal deaths. To determine the fetal death rate, the total number of intermediate and late fetal deaths (4) is divided by the total number of live births and the intermediate and late fetal deaths (100 + 4). The calculation is as follows:

$$\frac{(4 \times 100)}{(100 + 4)} = \frac{400}{104} = 3.846 = 3.85\%$$

Exercise 5.2

A hospital reported the following statistics for the month of April: live births, 500; newborn discharges, 510; intermediate fetal deaths, 2; and late fetal deaths, 3. Compute the fetal death rate for April. Carry out the answer to two decimal places.

Maternal Death Rate

A *maternal death* is defined as the death of any woman, from any cause, related to or aggravated by pregnancy or its management (regardless of duration or site of pregnancy, but not from accidental or incidental causes). The formula for calculating the maternal mortality rate is:

$$\frac{\textit{Number of direct maternal deaths for a period} \times 100}{\textit{Number of obstetrical discharges (including deaths) for the period}}$$

Healthcare facilities also differentiate between *direct* obstetric deaths and *indirect* obstetric deaths. The latter refers to deaths not directly due to obstetric causes, even though the physiologic effects of pregnancy are partially responsible for the death. When this rate is computed, hospitals usually classify only direct obstetric deaths as maternal deaths and include only those deaths that occur during hospitalization. Nonmaternal deaths (that is, deaths resulting from accidental or incidental causes not related to pregnancy or its management) are not included. A woman who dies after an abortion is a maternal death, as is an obstetrical patient who dies before delivery of a cause due to pregnancy. If the service classification system includes a breakdown of obstetrical discharges into delivered, aborted, not delivered, and postpartum admission services, all of these should be included in the total obstetrical discharges in the denominator of the formula (and in the numerator if they die).

For example, at one hospital a mother died immediately after delivery. The hospital's annual obstetric/gynecology discharges are classified as: delivered, 5,000; aborted, 100; not delivered (prepartum), 200; and not delivered (postpartum), 20.

The calculation of the hospital maternal mortality rate is:

$$\frac{(1 \times 100)}{(5{,}000 + 100 + 200 + 20)} = \frac{100}{5{,}320} = 0.0187 = 0.019\%$$

It is a good idea to carry this rate to three places beyond the decimal place because it is such a small number. Remember to use obstetrical discharges and not actual deliveries in the denominator.

As noted previously, researchers frequently use vital statistical information for public health and policy studies. The following vital statistics formula for maternal mortality rate may be used in the United States:

$$\frac{\textit{Number of deaths attributed to maternal conditions during a period} \times 100{,}000}{\textit{Number of live births during the period}}$$

For example, during the year, a women's hospital reported two deaths after abortions and 1,205 live births. The vital statistics maternal mortality rate is calculated as follows:

$$\frac{(2 \times 100{,}000)}{1{,}205} = \frac{200{,}000}{1{,}205} = 165.975 = 166 \textit{ per } 100{,}000 \textit{ births}$$

$$\frac{(2 \times 10{,}000)}{1{,}205} = \frac{20{,}000}{1{,}205} = 16.5975 = 16.6 \textit{ per } 10{,}000 \textit{ births}$$

$$\frac{(2 \times 1{,}000)}{1{,}205} = \frac{2{,}000}{1{,}205} = 1.65 = 1.7 \textit{ per } 1{,}000 \textit{ births}$$

Exercise 5.3

In the case of the women's hospital cited above, the obstetrical patients discharged included 50 aborted, 1,200 delivered, and 40 not delivered. Using the formula, calculate the hospital maternal mortality (death) rate. The hospital maternal mortality rate is 4 percent. True or false?

Cesarean Section Rate

As noted earlier, hospitals do not routinely calculate many of these rates. Raw data may be submitted to external agencies, which calculate the rate nationwide or by state, region, or locale. Hospitals may calculate these rates annually or only through special request. It may be necessary to report cesarean section rates to certain agencies such as the Joint Commission on Accreditation of Healthcare Organizations (JCAHO) or the American Medical Association (AMA) for such reasons as residency programs.

The formula for calculating the cesarean section rate is:

$$\frac{\textit{Total number of cesarean sections performed in a period} \times 100}{\textit{Total number of deliveries in the period (including cesarean sections)}}$$

Note that the cesarean section rate is not based on the number of patients discharged but, rather, on the number of deliveries. A rate compares the number of actual occurrences with the total possible; obviously, only deliveries can be cesarean sections. Usually, the data on deliveries and number of cesarean sections for the period are obtained from delivery room personnel.

For example, three cesarean sections were performed in a month during which there were 360 deliveries. The cesarean section rate is calculated by dividing the number of cesarean sections (3) by the total number of deliveries (360). The cesarean section rate is as follows:

$$\frac{(3 \times 100)}{360} = \frac{300}{360} = 0.833 = 0.83\%$$

Multiple births (that is, twins or triplets) constitute one delivery. Consequently, the number of births cannot be used for the formula.

Exercise 5.4

1. A women's hospital had 150 deliveries during June. Twins were born to three of the mothers. There were 169 obstetrical discharges. Cesarean sections were performed on two women. Calculate the cesarean section rate for June. The cesarean section rate for June is 1.33 percent. True or false?

2. Using data from an actual prenatal and infant care report below and the perinatal committee report in the infant mortality rate section of this chapter (see table 5.2), do the following:

   1. Validate the neonatal mortality rates within each weight category for 1994 using the vital statistics formula.

   2. Calculate the neonatal mortality rate for 1994.

   3. Calculate the hospital fetal death rate (more than 500 grams).

Prenatal and Infant Care Report

1/1/94–12/31/94

Birth Weight Grams	Fetal Deaths	Live Births	Neonatal Deaths
No Weight Available	1	0	0
≤ 500	4	10	7
501–749	2	7	4
750–999	0	10	0
1,000–1,499	3	26	2
1,500–1,999	3	52	0
2,000–2,499	3	167	2
2,500–2,999	1	556	1
3,000+	2	2,177	0
Total	**19**	**3,005**	**16**

Test on Obstetrical and Perinatal Rates

A hospital had the following statistics for the past year:

Discharges		Births (live)	1,615	Fetal Deaths	
Total adult and children	10,810			Intermediate	5
Total newborn	1,601	**Deaths**		Late	11
Obstetrical		Newborn	55		
Delivered	1,617	OB delivered	1		
Aborted	206	OB aborted	1		
Not delivered	109				

1. The hospital neonatal mortality rate is 3.44%.

    a. True
    b. False

2. The fetal death rate is:

    a. 0.98%
    b. 0.99%
    c. 1.00%
    d. None of the above

3. In computing the maternal mortality rate for the year, the formula would be interpreted as:

    a. $\dfrac{(2 \times 100)}{1,932}$

    b. $\dfrac{(2 \times 100)}{206}$

    c. $\dfrac{(1 \times 100)}{1,617}$

    d. $\dfrac{(2 \times 100)}{1,615}$

4. A hospital reports the following statistics for last year: births, 1,645; deliveries, 1,640; cesarean sections, 40; and obstetrical discharges, 1,932.

    The cesarean section rate for this year is:

    a. 2.04%
    b. 2.44%
    c. 2.43%
    d. 2.49%

Chapter 6
Morbidity and Other Rates

Objectives

At the conclusion of this chapter, you should be able to:

- Discuss infection rate
- Define and calculate postoperative infection rate
- Distinguish between a surgical procedure and a surgical operation
- Compute any other rate if provided with necessary data

Infection Rate

The term *morbidity* means the state of being diseased or the number of sick persons or cases of disease in relation to a specific population. Morbidity may be infectious or have other causes. For example, the presence of concomitant chronic conditions may constitute comorbidity. Moreover, morbidity may be preexisting or iatrogenic.

Preventing morbidity due to infection is an important quality management function. Frequently, the healthcare facility establishes a committee whose primary function is to evaluate infections and determine their causes so that recurrence can be avoided. Typically called the infection control committee, it is composed of representatives from the medical staff, nursing, pharmacy, risk management, and health information management. Charged with the duty of infection control, committee members establish procedures for the management and reporting of infections. Effective management of hospital infections sometimes requires finding cases beyond the infections listed by physicians on the face sheet. The HIM practitioner can help identify such cases in the course of performing qualitative analysis and/or coding processes.

As defined in chapter 1, rate refers to the number of times something occurred compared to the number of times it could have occurred. Each healthcare facility's medical staff must determine the criteria for inclusion in both numerator (infections) and denominator (patients at risk of infection). Most healthcare facilities differentiate between *nosocomial infections* (those acquired during hospitalization) and exacerbation or recurrence of previous infections. For example, if an obstetrical patient develops a urinary tract infection, a physician must determine whether it was hospital acquired or due to a recurrence of a previous urinary tract infection. In addition, the infection control committee determines whether acquired infections are attributable to specific patient care units (PCUs), specified operations, patients with specified diseases, the organized medical staff units, or individual physicians.

Infection rates may be calculated separately for specific infections such as surgical wound infections, puerperal infections, and infections of the respiratory tract, urinary tract, bloodstream, and so on. In addition to infections, healthcare facilities are concerned with any type of complication that results from, or occurs in, the course of care. Other types of complications that require special attention by medical staff and administration include wound disruptions, decubitus ulcers, postoperative hemorrhages, and adverse drug reactions. Specific infections or complications may be classified by their severity through the use of proprietary or public domain classification systems and compared to national norms.

Table 6.1 shows a report illustrating the severity of two conditions that, typically, are monitored by the hospital's infection control committee.

Postoperative Infection Rate

A *surgical procedure* is defined as any single, separate, systematic process upon or within the body that can be complete in itself; normally is performed by a physician, dentist, or other licensed practitioner; can be performed with or without instruments; and is performed to restore disunited or deficient parts, remove diseased or injured tissues, extract foreign matter, assist in obstetrical delivery, or aid in diagnosis. A *surgical operation* is defined as one or more surgical procedures performed at one time for one patient via a common

Table 6.1.   Report Showing Complications and Incisions and the Severity of Skin Ulcers and Gangrene

Fiscal Year 1997–1998

Disease Staging	Severity	Discharged	% Discharged	Average Length of Stay	Charge per Day
Complications of incisions	1.0	0	0	0	$0
	2.0	211	1.32	11.2	$1,159
	3.0	39	0.24	14.3	$1,679
	4.0	4	0.03	28.5	$2,553
Skin Ulcers and gangrene	1.0	32	0.20	31.5	$844
	2.0	33	0.21	30.2	$800
	3.0	5	0.03	73.8	$870
	4.0	0	0	0	0

approach or for a common purpose. An example of a surgical operation, including more than one surgical procedure, is an abdominoperineal resection. An example of two surgical operations and two surgical procedures is a tonsillectomy followed by a circumcision. Even though the procedures were performed at one time for one patient, the approach to each procedure is different and the two procedures are not for a common purpose.

The *postoperative infection rate* is the ratio of all infections in clean surgical cases to the number of surgical operations. Not all hospitals calculate this rate on a regular basis. The medical staff should provide guidance to the HIM practitioner and the infection control committee on what constitutes clean surgical cases. In addition, the hospital administration should decide how the postoperative infection rate is calculated (Huffman 1994). The formula for calculating this rate is:

$$\frac{Number\ of\ infections\ in\ clean\ surgical\ cases\ for\ a\ period \times 100}{Number\ of\ surgical\ operations\ for\ the\ period}$$

For example, during November, a hospital reported that 758 surgical operations were performed. The infection control committee reported one postoperative infection in a clean surgical case. According to the formula, the postoperative infection rate for November is calculated as follows:

$$\frac{(1 \times 100)}{758} = \frac{100}{758} = 0.1319 = 0.13\%$$

Other Rates

The HIM practitioner may compute and report other rates according to individual healthcare facility needs. External agencies also are asking that additional data and rates be reported. To pursue all the possibilities in this book is impractical. The best rule of thumb is to use the "other rates" formula. You may become so intrigued with this formula that you will volunteer to produce new and useful rates, which is, incidentally, part of your responsibility.

The formula for calculating other rates is:

$$\frac{Number\ of\ times\ something\ occurred \times 100}{Number\ of\ times\ something\ could\ have\ occurred}$$

It is important to remember that health records are a primary source of data used in compiling medical care statistics. Because HIM practitioners possess a broad range of knowledge about healthcare facilities and health record data, they are in the premium position to collect and prepare data as well as to analyze data and interpret them into statistical information.

However, statistics should not be kept just because they have always been kept. After you assure yourself, the administration, and the medical staff that a particular statistic no longer serves a useful purpose, stop keeping it. Do not be afraid to be creative and imaginative about providing new ideas for statistical computations that will serve a useful purpose, even if only on a temporary, special-study basis.

Exercise 6.1

Analyze the multi-hospital system statistical table on the next page, then respond to the following questions.

1. Which hospital has the lowest ALOS for incision complications at severity level 3?

2. Which hospital has the highest ALOS at severity level 3?

3. Which hospital has the highest charges per day for incision complications at severity level 3?

4. Which hospital has the least number of discharges for incision complications at severity level 3?

5. Which hospital has the highest number of discharges at severity level 3?

6. Which hospital has the highest charges per day for skin ulcer and gangrene at severity level 2?

7. Which hospital has the lowest ALOS for skin ulcer and gangrene at severity level 1?

8. Which hospital has the lowest charge per day for skin ulcer and gangrene at severity level 1?

9. Which hospital has the highest number of discharges for skin ulcer and gangrene at severity level 2?

Exercise 6.1 *(Continued)*

Fiscal Year 1997–1998

Conditions	Severity	Discharged	% Discharged	Average Length of Stay	Charge per Day
		Hospital A			
Complications of Incisions	1.0	0	0	0	0
	2.0	211	1.3	11.2	$1,159
	3.0	39	0.2	14.3	$1,679
	4.0	4	0	28.5	$2,553
Skin Ulcers and Gangrene	1.0	32	0.2	31.5	$844
	2.0	33	0.2	30.2	$800
	3.0	5	0	73.8	$870
	4.0	0	0	0	0
		Hospital B			
Complications of Incisions	1.0	0	0	0	0
	2.0	86	0.5	8.9	$1,563
	3.0	24	0.1	14.0	$1,579
	4.0	3	0	26.0	$2,485
Skin Ulcers and Gangrene	1.0	9	0.1	23.1	$1,111
	2.0	8	0	20.6	$1,288
	3.0	0	0	0	0
	4.0	0	0	0	0
		Hospital C			
Complications of Incisions	1.0	0	0	0	0
	2.0	342	1.5	9.5	$1,261
	3.0	145	0.6	14.3	$1,490
	4.0	13	0.1	32.2	$2,910
Skin Ulcers and Gangrene	1.0	15	0.1	16.1	$947
	2.0	42	0.2	14.5	$1,159
	3.0	1	0	20.0	$1,221
	4.0	0	0	0	0
		Hospital D			
Complications of Incisions	1.0	0	0	0	0
	2.0	168	0.8	11.3	$1,049
	3.0	36	0.2	18.1	$1,144
	4.0	0	0	0	0
Skin Ulcers and Gangrene	1.0	11	0.1	21.1	$641
	2.0	22	0.1	17.3	$1,147
	3.0	0	0	0	0
	4.0	0	0	0	0

Test on Morbidity and Other Rates

Complete sections A and B.

Section A

1. Each healthcare facility must keep infection rates for each medical care unit.

   a. True
   b. False

2. There are specific, generally accepted criteria to be included in the formula for hospital infection rate.

   a. True
   b. False

3. A nosocomial infection is one that was acquired during hospitalization.

   a. True
   b. False

4. The postoperative infection rate is the ratio of all infections in clean surgical cases to the number of surgical procedures.

   a. True
   b. False

Section B

A hospital reported the following annual statistics:

Total adult and children discharges	10,810
Total newborn discharges	1,601
Surgical procedures	1,010
Surgical operations	1,005
Patients receiving consultations	2,013
Hospital-incurred infections	11

1. The hospital infection rate (including newborns) is:

   a. 0.09%
   b. 0.10%
   c. 1.10%
   d. None of the above

2. What is the consultation rate (including newborns)?

   a. 16.4%
   b. 16.2%
   c. 18.6%
   d. None of the above

Chapter 7
Death (Mortality) Rates

Objectives

At the conclusion of this chapter, you should be able to:

- Define and calculate death rate
- Discuss net death rate, postoperative death rate, and anesthesia death rate
- Calculate postoperative death rate
- Define cancer mortality rate

Death Rate

The hospital *death rate* is the proportion of inpatient hospitalizations that end in death, usually expressed as a percentage. A synonymous term for hospital death rate is *gross death rate*.

Death rates have always been important information for health agencies and hospitals in evaluating the quality of medical care. For example, in 1991, the New York State Health Department used them to rank the state's cardiovascular surgeons and their performance. According to a September 8, 1995, article in the *New York Times,* these mortality rates eventually forced 21 of the low-ranking doctors out of their specialty in New York. Lives were saved in one hospital when the same statistical ranking provoked a reengineering of patient care methods that applied state standards more strictly to caring for patients before heart surgery. HIM practitioners—and anyone else who relies on statistical information—must always remember that numbers count, not only in reports and records, but also in the human equation.

Death rate data also have been important in helping public health agencies plan for health services. For example, the Health Care Financing Administration (HCFA) previously published a report for each hospital on Medicare deaths. Initially, HCFA mortality data received a great deal of media coverage and caused concern in facilities because of the high percentages reported. In addition, the report created confusion about definitions and interpretation of the data. Hospitals were permitted to correct the data, and since the initial releases, HCFA has modified the report format. This demonstrates the importance of the HIM practitioner's need to comprehend death rates. HIM practitioners must understand basic death rates and be ready to calculate or verify other data pertaining to mortality.

Formula for Calculating Death Rate

In calculating hospital death rate, the concept of number of occurrences versus number of times something could have occurred still applies. That is, every patient discharged from the hospital could possibly have died. Of course, this does not happen, but it is still a statistical possibility. Therefore, the formula for calculating hospital death rate is the number of patient deaths divided by the number of patient discharges (including deaths), as shown below:

$$\frac{\textit{Number of inpatient deaths in a period} \times 100}{\textit{Number of discharges (including deaths) in the period}}$$

For example, if a hospital had 5 deaths and 400 discharges for a month, the gross death rate is:

$$\frac{(5 \times 100)}{400} = 1.25\%$$

Guidelines for Calculating Death Rate

Death rate is one of the rates that HIM practitioners calculate on the job every day. In calculating hospital death rate, the following guidelines should be considered:

- Death is a type of discharge. Any data representing total discharges include deaths for that period. Thus, deaths are always assumed to be included in the total discharges in the denominator.

- If deaths of newborn inpatients are included in the numerator, all discharges of newborn inpatients must be included in the denominator.

- Patients who are dead on arrival (DOA) are not included in the hospital inpatient death rate because DOAs are not admitted to the hospital.

- Patients who die in the ED are not included in the hospital inpatient death rate because they were not admitted to the hospital.

- Fetal deaths are not included in the hospital death rate but, rather, are usually calculated separately.

- Because death rates are fairly small, the calculation should be carried out to at least two decimal places.

- It is a good idea to put a zero in front of the decimal (for example, 0.23%) to show the casual observer that the rate is less than one percent.

Exercise 7.1

Using the data below, calculate the gross death rate for June.

Total adults and children discharges	600
Total adults and children deaths	3
Total newborn discharges	90
Total newborn deaths	1

Other, Specific Death Rate Data

As discussed in chapter 5, hospitals may calculate fetal death rate, infant mortality rate, and maternal death rate. They also may choose to calculate net death rate, postoperative death rate, and anesthesia death rate.

Net Death Rate

The *net death rate* is sometimes requested by various reporting or accrediting agencies. Previously, hospital inpatient deaths were classified by the period elapsed from the time of admission, according to whether they occurred within 48 hours of, or more than 48 hours after, admission. The net death rate excludes deaths under 48 hours and is smaller than the gross death rate.

Basically, the net death rate was an adjustment made to recognize that healthcare providers should not be accountable for death that occurs during the early hours of a patient's stay because they would not have had enough time to directly affect the patient's condition. However, with the technology available today, many authorities believe this concept is no longer valid.

Postoperative Death Rate

Postoperative death rate refers to the number of deaths occurring after an operation has been performed. Standard instructions for computing postoperative death rate involve the ratio of deaths within ten days after surgery to the total number of operations performed during the period.

However, some healthcare practitioners question the usefulness of this calculation in evaluating the effectiveness of a hospital's medical care. Thus, rather than compute a total postoperative death rate, some hospitals evaluate the relationship of deaths following specific operations (for example, cholecystectomies or coronary artery bypass grafts).

Anesthesia Death Rate

The traditional definition of *anesthesia death rate* is the ratio of deaths caused by anesthetic agents during a period to the number of anesthetics administered. Because anesthesia deaths occur infrequently, some hospitals might choose, instead, to evaluate the relationship between a death and a specific anesthetic for a special study.

Cancer Mortality Rate

A mortality rate measures the risk of death for the cause under study in a defined population during a given time period. For cancer, the National Center for Health Statistics collects data on all deaths occurring in the United States and classifies them by sex, age, race, and cancer site so that mortality for a given time period can be determined for the entire country or selected areas.

The formula for calculating the cancer mortality rate is:

$$\frac{\textit{Number of cancer deaths during a period} \times 100,000}{\textit{Total number in population at risk}}$$

In 1987, for example, 476,927 people died from cancer in the United States. The midyear population in the U.S. was estimated to be 243,394,693. Using the cancer mortality rate formula, the cancer mortality (death) rate per 100,000 for the U.S. in 1987 was:

$$\frac{\textit{Number of cancer deaths in 1987} \times 100,000}{\textit{Population at risk}}$$

$$\frac{(476,927 \times 100,000)}{243,394,693} = 195.9 \textit{ deaths per } 100,000 \textit{ population}$$

This is a crude death rate because it encompasses deaths from all forms of cancer for persons of all ages and races and of both sexes; that is, it is based on the entire U.S. population. Specific rates may be calculated to describe risks for specific cancers in entire populations or specific subgroups of a population, such as age-specific rates or sex-specific rates (SEER Program 1994).

For example, according to a report titled *Cancer Incidence and Mortality by Race/ Ethnicity in California, 1988–1991* (State of California 1994), breast cancer accounted for more than a quarter (28.3 percent) of all cancer diagnoses in women, making it the most commonly diagnosed cancer among women in all four race/ethnic groups. It was the second leading cause of cancer-related mortality among Asian/other, non-Hispanic black, and non-Hispanic white women, and the leading cause of death due to cancer in Hispanic women. Lung cancer accounted for 15 percent of all cancer diagnoses and 27.1 percent of all cancer-related mortality. It was the leading cause of cancer mortality among all sex and race/ethnic groups except Hispanic females.

Knowledge of healthcare statistics is an essential tool for tumor (cancer) registrars. Cancer registry data are reported by hospitals to population-based (central) registries. Hospital cancer programs publish a cancer annual report and statistical review that is required by the American College of Surgeons for approved programs.

Exercise 7.2

Using the following statistics from an actual report published by a multihospital system, validate the death rate for each hospital listed and for the entire healthcare system.

XYZ Healthcare System
Fiscal Year 1994 Statistics

Hospital	Discharges	Deaths	Death Rate
1	18,114	280	1.55%
2	19,552	207	1.06%
3	4,857	83	1.71%
4	2,737	41	1.50%
Total System	**45,260**	**611**	**1.35%**

Test on Death (Mortality) Rates

Complete sections A and B.

Section A

Using the data reported by one hospital for the past year, perform the calculations requested below.

Discharges		Deaths	
Total adults and children	10,810	Total adults and children	40
Total newborns	1,601	Total newborns	3
		Within 10 days postoperative	2
Admissions			
Total adults and children	10,850		
Total births	1,615	Total operations	3,975

1. The hospital death rate is:

   a. 0.035%
   b. 0.37%
   c. 0.346%
   d. 0.037%

2. The postoperative death rate is 0.05 percent.

   a. True
   b. False

Section B

Select the best answer to the following questions:

1. The gross death rate excludes deaths that occur within 48 hours of admission.

   a. True
   b. False

2. According to standard instructions, deaths within fifteen days after surgery are used to compute the postoperative death rate.

   a. True
   b. False

3. Anesthesia deaths occur frequently.

   a. True
   b. False

Chapter 8
Hospital Autopsies and Autopsy Rates

Objectives

At the conclusion of this chapter, you should be able to:

- Define the terms *hospital inpatient autopsy, hospital autopsy,* and *autopsy rate*
- Compute gross autopsy rate
- Compute net autopsy rate
- Compute adjusted hospital autopsy rate

Gross Autopsy Rate

An *autopsy rate* is the proportion of deaths that are followed by the performance of an autopsy. *Gross autopsy rate* is the ratio during any given period of time of all inpatient autopsies to all inpatient deaths. The rate is customarily reported as a percentage. Again, the concept of the number of times something occurred to the number of times it could have occurred applies. Statistically speaking, every patient who dies could be autopsied. Typically, newborn deaths and autopsies are included in the gross autopsy rate.

The formula for calculating gross autopsy rate is:

$$\frac{Total\ inpatient\ autopsies\ for\ a\ period \times 100}{Total\ inpatient\ deaths\ for\ the\ period}$$

For example, during July, a hospital discharged 918 patients. The hospital had 32 deaths (including newborns) and performed 9 autopsies. Using the formula given above, the gross autopsy rate is determined to be 28.13 percent, as follows:

$$\frac{(9 \times 100)}{32} = \frac{900}{32} = 28.125 = 28.13\%$$

Although death rates are small, autopsy rates can be fairly large.

Exercise 8.1

During a one-month period, a 360-bed hospital with 20 bassinets reported 38 inpatient deaths. The medical staff performed 12 autopsies. The gross autopsy rate is 31.58 percent. True or false?

Net Autopsy Rate

Net autopsy rate is the ratio during any given period of time of all inpatient autopsies to all inpatient deaths, minus unautopsied coroners' or medical examiners' cases. The formula for net autopsy rate differs slightly from the one for gross autopsy rate in that it excludes coroners' or medical examiners' cases that are not autopsied at the hospital.

The formula for calculating net autopsy rate is:

$$\frac{Total\ inpatient\ autopsies\ for\ a\ period \times 100}{Total\ inpatient\ deaths - Unautopsied\ coroners'\ or\ medical\ examiners'\ cases}$$

For example, during August, a hospital had 42 patient deaths and performed 14 autopsies. Two bodies were released to the county coroner for autopsy. Therefore, two cases are subtracted from the denominator because they were not autopsied by the hospital. Dividing the number of inpatient autopsies performed (14) by the total number of bodies available for autopsy ($42 - 2 = 40$) produces a net autopsy rate of 35 percent.

$$\frac{(14 \times 100)}{(42 - 2)} = \frac{1,400}{40} = 35.0\%$$

Exercise 8.2

A hospital had 630 discharges, 14 inpatient deaths, and 11 autopsies during May. Two deaths were unavailable for autopsy because they were released to the medical examiner. What is the net autopsy rate for this hospital?

Hospital Autopsies

A *hospital inpatient autopsy* is the postmortem examination performed in a hospital facility on the body of an inpatient who died during hospitalization. In contrast, a *hospital autopsy* is the postmortem examination, wherever performed, of the body of a person who has *at some time* been a hospital patient. In both cases, the autopsy is performed by a staff pathologist or a physician delegated to perform it in place of a pathologist.

When determining what autopsies should be included in the hospital autopsy rate, the following guidelines apply:

- Usually, hospital autopsies are performed by the staff pathologist. However, small hospitals do not always have a pathologist on staff, so responsibility for performing autopsies is delegated to another physician.

- Normally, hospital autopsies are performed in hospitals. However, a small hospital or a specialized (for example, obstetrical) hospital may not have many deaths and thus may not have the necessary facilities to perform autopsies. In such cases, the autopsies are performed in another designated place.

- As a general rule, hospital autopsies are performed on deceased inpatients. However, because of the educational value of autopsies, previous patients who are not in the hospital at the time of death may be considered for hospital autopsies.

- Fetal autopsies are not included in the hospital autopsy rate because a fetus is not considered a patient.

- The essentials of a hospital autopsy are:

    —The autopsy must be performed by a staff pathologist or a delegated physician.

    —The autopsy report must be filed in the patient's health record.

    —The tissue specimens must be filed in the hospital laboratory along with the autopsy report.

Examples of hospital autopsies include:

- A patient dies in the hospital and is autopsied by the hospital's pathologist in the local morgue.

- A patient dies in the hospital and one of the hospital's doctors is delegated to perform the autopsy in the absence of the staff pathologist.

- A patient is pronounced DOA in the hospital's ED where he had been discharged three months earlier, and an autopsy is performed by the staff pathologist.

Adjusted Hospital Autopsy Rate

Adjusted hospital autopsy rate is the proportion of hospital autopsies performed following the deaths of patients whose bodies are available for autopsy. Although many hospitals calculate the net autopsy rate for various surveys and external reports, the adjusted hospital autopsy rate is a more accurate indication of the hospital's resources for physician education.

The formula for calculating adjusted hospital autopsy rate is:

$$\frac{Total\ hospital\ autopsies \times 100}{Total\ number\ of\ deaths\ of\ hospital\ patients\ whose\ bodies\ are\ available\ for\ hospital\ autopsy}$$

Patients whose bodies are available for hospital autopsy include:

- Inpatients (unless the bodies are removed from the hospital by legal authorities such as coroners, medical examiners, or anatomical boards). However, if the hospital pathologist or delegated physician performs an autopsy while acting as an agent of the coroner, the autopsy is included in the numerator and the death in the denominator of the adjusted hospital autopsy rate formula.

- Other patients, including hospital home care patients, outpatients, and previous hospital patients who have died elsewhere whose bodies have been made available for the performance of hospital autopsies.

The tenth edition of *Health Information Management* (Huffman 1994) gives the following example:

During [the month of] September 25 inpatient deaths occurred. Among these [deaths were] 3 deaths that had to be reported to the coroner; 2 of these bodies were removed from the hospital so no hospital autopsy was performed; 1 hospital autopsy was performed on the other case. This was 1 of the 15 hospital autopsies performed following the inpatient deaths during the month. In addition to the 15 autopsies performed on inpatient deaths, hospital autopsies were also performed on 16 outpatients who were former inpatients]. . . . Therefore, these 6 deaths are added to the 25 available inpatient deaths and the 6 additional hospital autopsies are counted. The adjusted hospital autopsy rate is computed as follows:

$$\frac{(15 + 6) \times 100}{25 + 6 - 2} = \frac{2,100}{29} = 72.41\%$$

This adjusted hospital autopsy rate . . . truly gives an accurate picture of the service rendered by the hospital pathologist for teaching and scientific purposes . . . (Huffman 1994, 421).

Exercise 8.3

In August, a hospital had 38 inpatient deaths, 12 of which were autopsied. Of the 38 deaths, three were coroners' cases: one was autopsied by the hospital patholo-gist, and two were removed without autopsy. Moreover, the following cases were brought to the hospital to be autopsied: a former inpatient who died in a skilled nursing facility a month after discharge from the hospital; a child known to have congenital heart disease who died in the ED; and a former inpatient who died at home while under hospital home care. What is the adjusted hospital autopsy rate for this hospital?

Test on Hospital Autopsies and Autopsy Rates

Complete sections A and B.

Section A

Last year, a hospital reported the following statistics:

Inpatient discharges

Total adults and children	10,810
Total newborns	1,601
Total inpatient discharges	*12,411*

Inpatient deaths

Total adults and children	40
Total newborns	3
Total inpatient deaths	*43*
Total inpatient autopsies	38
Unautopsied coroners' cases	2
Hospital autopsied outpatients	2

Select the data needed from the above statistics to calculate the following:

1. Gross autopsy rate:

    a. 95.0%
    b. 88.37%
    c. 0.37%
    d. 0.19%

2. Net autopsy rate:

   a. 92.68%
   b. 87.80%
   c. 88.37%
   d. 9.29%

3. Adjusted hospital autopsy rate:

   a. 92.68%
   b. 88.37%
   c. 93.02%
   d. 97.56%

Section B

1. Which of the following represents a hospital autopsy? List as many letters as apply:

   a. A former inpatient died at home a month after discharge from the hospital, and his body was brought to the hospital for autopsy.

   b. The hospital pathologist was authorized by the coroner to perform an autopsy on a patient who died in the ED after a car accident.

   c. A patient who had been receiving radiation therapy on an outpatient basis at the hospital died at home; her body was brought to the hospital for autopsy.

   d. A victim of gunshot wounds who died in the ED was autopsied by the medical examiner.

   e. A cardiac patient died in the ED, and the hospital pathologist performed the autopsy.

   f. The hospital pathologist designated a physician to cover for her while she was away. The physician performed an autopsy on a deceased hospital inpatient.

   g. A late fetal death (stillbirth) was autopsied by the hospital pathologist.

2. What is the principal difference between net autopsy rate and adjusted hospital autopsy rate?

   a. Fetal deaths are not counted in hospital autopsy rates.

   b. Hospital autopsy rates include only those deaths where the bodies are available for autopsy.

   c. Net autopsy rate considers only inpatient deaths.

   d. Legal cases sometimes are excluded from deaths when computing net autopsy rate.

Test on Chapters 7 and 8

Complete sections A and B.

Section A

The following statistical data were reported by a hospital for April 1999:

Discharges
Total adults and children	903
Total newborns	149
Total inpatient discharges	*1,052*

Deaths
Total adults and children	19
Total newborns	5
Total inpatient deaths	*24*
Fetal deaths	9

Autopsies
Total adults and children	14
Total newborns	4
Total inpatient autopsies	*18*
Hospital autopsied outpatients	3
Unautopsied coroners' cases	2

Using data from the statistics above, write the formula you would use to calculate the following rates:

Example: Newborn death rate: $\dfrac{(5 \times 100)}{149}$

1. Death rate

2. Gross autopsy rate

3. Net autopsy rate

4. Adjusted hospital autopsy rate

Section B

Indicate whether each of the following statements is true or false:

1. To be considered a hospital autopsy, the autopsy must be performed by the staff pathologist or a physician delegated the responsibility.

2. A hospital autopsy must be performed in the hospital.

3. Hospital autopsies are performed only on inpatients.

4. Autopsies on fetuses are included in hospital autopsies.

5. The essentials of a hospital autopsy are that it be performed by the hospital pathologist or a physician delegated the responsibility, that an autopsy report be filed in the patient's health record, and that tissue specimens and the autopsy report be filed in the hospital laboratory.

6. Net autopsy rate includes both inpatients and out-of-hospital patients.

7. A deceased hospital inpatient whose body is released to legal authorities for autopsy is not included in computing net autopsy rate.

Chapter 9
Statistics Computed within the Health Information Management Department

Objectives

At the conclusion of this chapter, you should be able to:

- Describe the uses of statistics computed within the HIM department
- Determine how to calculate effective medical transcription unit labor costs
- Calculate cost breakdown of release of information requests
- Explain some of the measures used within the HIM department to determine staff workload levels
- Recognize how statistics are used within the HIM department to plan work space and health record storage

Staff Workload and Productivity

Statistics computed for use within the HIM department usually relate to staff workload and productivity and often are used in determining new hires, setting benchmarks for productivity, and so on. The following sections provide examples of common, everyday computations made by HIM staff members.

Medical Transcription

Effective transcription management decisions require accurate and complete information about the HIM department and its staff. Two elements that are key to determining effective transcription management are transcriptionist compensation and unit workload. Statistics on compensation and workload are calculated as follows:

- *Annual compensation for each medical transcriptionist:* The annual compensation for an individual transcriptionist is calculated by multiplying the number of hours worked per year (2,088 for a full-time employee) by the hourly wage and then multiplying that number by the benefits received. For example:

$$2,088 \text{ } hours \times \$10 \text{ } per \text{ } hour \times 1.3 \text{ } (30\% \text{ } benefits) = \$27,144.$$

- *Unit medical transcription labor cost:* Transcription workload is commonly measured in lines or minutes of work added to the system and transcribed by the staff. To determine unit transcription labor cost, divide the total transcriptionist annual compensation by total annual productivity, as shown below:

$$\frac{Total \text{ } (sum) \text{ } medical \text{ } transcriptionist \text{ } annual \text{ } compensation}{Total \text{ } (sum) \text{ } medical \text{ } transcriptionist \text{ } annual \text{ } productivity} = \$/unit$$

For example:

2 full-time employees produce 900 lines:	1 makes $7.50 per hour
	1 makes $8.00 per hour
5 full-time employees produce 1,000 lines:	1 makes $8.00 per hour
	3 make $8.50 per hour
	1 makes $9.00 per hour
2 full-time employees produce 1,100 lines:	1 makes $9.00 per hour
	1 makes $9.50 per hour
1 full-time employee produces 1,200 lines:	1 makes $10.00 per hour

Annual compensation:

1 full-time employee at $7.50 per hour	= $20,358 per year
2 full-time employees at $8.00 per hour	= $43,430 per year
3 full-time employees at $8.50 per hour	= $71,106 per year
2 full-time employees at $9.00 per hour	= $48,860 per year
1 full-time employee at $9.50 per hour	= $25,787 per year
1 full-time employee at $10.00 per hour	= $27,144 per year
Total:	**$236,685 per year**

Annual productivity:

2 full-time employees transcribed 900 lines   =   437,400 lines per year
5 full-time employees transcribed 1,000 lines = 1,215,000 lines per year
2 full-time employees transcribed 1,100 lines =   534,600 lines per year
1 full-time employee transcribed 1,200 lines =   291,600 lines per year

Total: **2,478,600 lines per year**

$$\frac{\$236,685}{2,478,600 \ lines} = \$0.0955 \ (approximately \ 9^1/_2 \ cents \ per \ line)$$

Exercise 9.1

1. What is the unit medical transcription labor cost for the full-time employee who provides 1,200 lines?

2. What is the unit medical transcription labor cost for the full-time employee who makes $8.50 per hour?

Release of Information Cost Breakdown

To justify costs for *correspondence copying* for health record services, one HIM professional needed to calculate cost breakdowns according to the following examples:

Average requests per month = 737

Postage:
$553 per month in postage costs $= \dfrac{\$553}{737} = \$0.75$ per request

Service:
$116 per month for copier and microfilm reader/printer $= \dfrac{\$116}{737} = \$0.16$ per request

Equipment:
$164 per month for copier and microfilm reader/printer accumulated depreciation expense $= \dfrac{\$164}{737} = \$0.22$ per request

Supplies:
$66 per month for cost of toner, printer ribbons, copy paper, and envelopes $= \dfrac{\$66}{737} = \$0.09$ per request

Work space:
Total of 97 sq. ft. used for ROI purposes. Reconstruction costs are $253 per sq. ft. for a total cost of $24,541 depreciated at 15% per year. $= \$3,681$ cost of space per year $= \$307$ per 737 requests $= \dfrac{\$307}{737}$ $= \$0.42$ per request

Total cost of postage, service, equipment, supplies, and work space: $1.64 per request.

Exercise 9.2

Calculate the cost breakdown for an HIM department receiving the following per month averages:

Requests	532	Equipment	$158
Postage	$482	Supplies	$72
Service	$128	Work space	$313

Patient Record Processing

Processing patient record (chart) requests consumes a great deal of HIM staff time. Responsibilities in maintaining charts include:

- *Chart pulls:* If the department uses a computerized tracking system, reports may be generated that display the number of chart pulls each month based on reason for request, requestor or department in which the requestor is located (chart tracking location), or charts requested as "stat" versus "routine" requests. In manually tracked statistics, the requests may only reflect the number of requests, or time needed, although those for prescheduled appointments (which are received separately from other requests) may be tracked separately.

- *New charts:* The department generally tracks the number of new charts (chart folders set up for new patients) created each month. However, this may not tally with statistics on new patients that are generated from a practice management system. The definition of the term *new patient* in a practice management system relies on the *CPT-4* code definition of new versus established patient. A chart already may exist for a patient that can be considered "new" to an individual provider or department.

- *Loose papers:* The number of pieces of paper received in the HIM department for filing is a significant factor in determining staffing levels. Loose papers may be measured in inches or by individual pieces, which is a more accurate measure. Because of the time involved in tracking this information, departments may choose to sample this activity for a one-week period several times a year.

- *Active/inactive charts:* Often charts that are considered inactive (no patient contact with the facility) are stored in a separate location from the main HIM file room. Their location and the definition of inactive status may have more to do with storage space in the main file room than actual inactivity. The workload associated with inactive charts is different from that associated with active charts being pulled and refiled and having loose papers added to them. However, inactive charts may require more resources when charts are needed because they are less accessible than charts in the main file room.

- *Chart availability:* The percentage of charts available at the time they are needed, or the average time it takes to provide a chart to fill a request, are important indicators to providers and the management of HIM department effectiveness.

Maintaining this information can be cumbersome if the department does not use a computerized tracking system. With a manual system, the information may be limited to how many charts needed for prescheduled appointments for each provider were available (pulled and forwarded to the provider) prior to the day of the appointment. With a computerized system, however, it may be possible to generate reports showing the actual turnaround time based on type of request and to determine the percentage that is delivered within whatever chart availability standards have been set by the organization. This can be further analyzed by categorizing turnaround based on whether the chart was in file at the time of the request or needed to be obtained from another location. (Optical disk storage is discussed in a later section of this chapter.)

Figure 9.1 shows an actual report of time allocation in an HIM department. This detailed report shows the hours spent on processing patient records. The time allocations are differentiated for the processing of various types of patient records, including ED, general clinic, outpatient/ambulatory surgery, and inpatient. Then the inpatient total hours are differentiated by service categories: pediatrics, OB/AB, psychiatric, NB, and med/surg.

Additional General Responsibilities

In addition to the chart responsibilities above, HIM staff time is used in performing the following activities:

- *Fielding telephone calls:* It is helpful to know how many calls are being received and at what time of day in order to determine staffing coverage. Usually, these statistics are kept manually, often in the form of a "tick" sheet showing day of week and time of day.

- *Releasing records:* If the release of information (ROI) function is centralized within the HIM department, requests for copies of medical records usually are tracked, and often counted, based on reason for the request (ongoing medical care, referral to another provider, attending physician statement) or type of requestor (attorney, insurance company, patient). This information can be used to help the facility plan marketing campaigns, staff recruitment, and so on. For example, the facility may want to know how many patients are leaving the practice for another physician or group. To obtain this information, the facility may hold patient satisfaction (exit) interviews based on information provided by HIM to determine why patients are choosing other health care providers.

Ratios for Determining Staffing Levels in Departments in Which Functions Are Separated

If the HIM department is large enough to separate job duties such as ROI and transcription support, these staff may need to be counted separately for purposes of determining staffing levels. Moreover, this would be true if some functions are centralized (for example, a separate ROI department/section of HIM may process ROIs for all of the satellites/branches of a large clinic). Common ratios generated include:

- *Encounters per FTE per month:* This is determined by dividing the number of patient encounters by the number of staff. FTEs may be determined from payroll reports based on hours worked, hours paid, or budgeted positions for the period. A decision needs to be made as to whether some patient encounters at the facility

Figure 9.1   Health Information Services Time Allocation Report, September 1999

		Hours
Emergency Department Records		
Clerical:	Processing (28 h/w × 4.3 weeks)	120.4
Correspondence:	(7 h/w × 4.3 weeks)	30.1
Supervisory:	(5 h/w × 4.3 weeks)	21.5
General Clinic		
Clerical:	Processing (6 h/w × 4.3 weeks)	25.8
Supervisory:	(.5 h/w × 4.3 weeks)	2.2
Transcription:	(.1033 h/record × 170)	17.6
Outpatient/Ambulatory Surgery—All Categories		
Clerical:	Primary	86.0
	Filing	21.5
	Admissions	10.8
	Combining	4.3
	Tumor Registry	4.3
	Correspondence	1.1
	Record Completion	43.0
	Certificates	12.9
Supervisory:	(5 h/w × 4.3 weeks)	21.5
Transcription:	(.1033 h/record × 627.9)	64.9
Coding:	(.0833 h/record × 897)	74.7
Inpatient Records		
Total Hours Paid		4941.4
Minus Emergency, Clinic, Outpatient Hours		562.5
Inpatient Total Hours		4378.9
Pediatrics		47.6
OB/AB		238.2
Psychiatric		394.1
NB		203.6
Med/Surg		3495.3
Percentage Distribution Categories		
Emergency Department		3.5
Clinic		0.9
OPT/AMB SURG		7.0
Pediatrics		1.0
OB/AB		4.8
Psychiatry		8.0
NB		4.1
Med/Surg		70.7
	Total	**100.0**

Prepared by XXXXXXXXXXX, Director, Health Information Services
Date: 10/23/99

should be included when determining HIM staff ratios. For example, the HIM department may not routinely pull charts for an urgency care center but still have responsibility for assigning a medical record number and setting up a chart for the record. A weighting factor might be assigned to urgency care visits, indicating that less HIM staff time is required to support this encounter. Laboratory, radiology, and other ancillary departments may be included or excluded from the total patient encounters for HIM purposes, especially if charts are not routinely pulled for these encounters. A more accurate measure of the workload generated for HIM staff from laboratory or radiology may be the number of tests or the number of reports if more than one test is reported on a single piece of paper.

- *Providers per FTE per month:* Again, some adjustment may need to be made to the count maintained by the medical staff office, based on the support required from HIM.

- *Charts per FTE:* This is determined by dividing the total number of charts maintained in the file room by the number of FTEs in the HIM department. Inactive records may be given a weighted value (for example, one inactive chart equals one-third of an active chart) in this calculation.

Work Space

In addition to determining workload and staffing level, statistics computed within the HIM department may be useful in planning work space. For example, file room space or shelving needs may be estimated by dividing file room growth by the average number of charts per foot of file shelving. File room growth is determined by adding the number of new charts added each month/year to the expansion in size of existing charts based on inches of loose papers received each month/year minus the number of charts that are likely to become inactive during the month/year. The average number of charts per foot of shelf space is determined by counting the number of charts in twelve inches of shelving at random locations throughout the file room.

Optical Disk Storage

When evaluating the feasibility of optical disk storage, several elements must be examined. First, you must know the number of bytes of the optical disk platter in question. To review:

- 1 kilobyte = 1,000 bytes
- 1 megabyte = 1,000,000 bytes
- 1 gigabyte = 1,000,000,000 bytes

Current densities of optical disk platters vary. Twelve-inch platters store approximately 5.6 gigabytes, and $5\frac{1}{4}$-inch platters store approximately 1.3 gigabytes.

Second, to determine the number of pages per platter, you must know the density of the document in question. This varies greatly depending on the document. Forms, letters, and rhythm strips all vary in the number of light and dark dots per page. Scanned images take up many more bytes than images that have been interfaced from another system electronically. The usual approximation is that a letter is usually 30 to 50 kilobytes (K) and an average document is approximately 70K or 70,000 bytes.

For example, using a 5.6-gigabyte platter and an image size of 70K, you would be able to store 80,000 pages per platter, as shown below:

$$\frac{5,600,000,000}{70,000} = 80,000$$

Exercise 9.3

1. Interview a health information professional to learn what statistical calculations he or she uses on the job. Report your findings to the class.

2. Using the information in the time allocation report below, complete these exercises:

    • Discuss in class what changes you would make to the report for clarification purposes, for presentation effect, and so on.

    • With class members, brainstorm possible uses for this report, its audience or potential viewers, or the delineations of patient records.

Health Information Services
Time Allocation Report—September 1999

		Hours
Emergency Department Records		
Clerical:	Processing (28 h/w × 4.3 weeks)	120.4
Correspondence:	(7 h/w × 4.3 weeks)	30.1
Supervisory:	(5 h/w × 4.3 weeks)	21.5
General Clinic		
Clerical:	Processing (6 h/w × 4.3 weeks)	25.8
Supervisory:	(.5 h/w × 4.3 weeks)	2.2
Transcription:	(.1033 h/record × 170)	17.6
Outpatient/Ambulatory Surgery – All Categories		
Clerical:	Primary	86.0
	Filing	21.5
	Admissions	10.8
	Combining	4.3
	Tumor Registry	4.3
	Correspondence	1.1
	Record Completion	43.0
	Certificates	12.9
Supervisory:	(5 h/w × 4.3 weeks)	21.5
Transcription:	(.1033 h/record × 627.9)	64.9
Coding:	(.0833 h/record × 897)	74.7

Exercise 9.3 *(Continued)*

Inpatient Records	
Total Hours Paid	4941.4
Minus Emergency, Clinic, Outpatient Hours	562.5
Inpatient Total Hours	4378.9
Pediatrics	47.6
OB/AB	238.2
Psychiatric	394.1
NB	203.6
Med/Surg	3495.3
Percentage Distribution Categories	
Emergency Department	3.5
Clinic	0.9
OPT/AMB SURG	7.0
Pediatrics	1.0
OB/AB	4.8
Psychiatry	8.0
NB	4.1
Med/Surg	70.7
Total	**100.0**

Prepared by XXXXXXXXXXX, Director, Health Information Services
Date: 10/23/99

Chapter 10
Statistics Computed for Alternative Care Settings

Objectives

At the conclusion of this chapter, you should be able to:

- Calculate resource allocation in managed care organizations
- Discuss the types of statistics kept for ambulatory care facilities
- Recognize how long-term care statistics may differ from traditional acute care statistics
- Describe two instruments used to calculate statistics in behavioral (mental) health settings

Managed Care Organizations

Resource allocation in most managed care organizations (MCOs) is done by member months or per member per month (PMPM). If the MCO provides care to high-risk groups such as Medicare or Medicaid patients, the PMPM figures are normally weighted to account for their higher utilization levels. The weighting factors are MCO specific. The process of weighting is referred to as *calculating adjusted member months.* Most calculations are made using 1,000 member months or 1,000 adjusted member months as the basis.

Use of Adjusted Member Months

The *projected member months,* or the number of members that will be served in the coming month, are provided by the enrollment department by the fifteenth of the month. These figures are used in calculating allowable staffing levels in patient care departments. To determine this staffing level, the adjusted member months must be divided by 1,000 and then multiplied by the staffing factor for the department. The use of adjusted member months accounts for the increased numbers of visits and services generated by a particular mix of high-risk groups.

Expected levels of laboratory tests, X-ray exams, or other services also can be estimated from adjusted member months to allow proper supply budgeting, as well as staff, to perform the labor. The estimation process is referred to as *estimating PMPM* or *budgeting PMPM.* Actual levels of performance or utilization are calculated based on member months and compared to the budget calculations to determine budget variance. If necessary, the next budget year would use a revised staffing or supply ratio.

Bed Days as a Standard Measure of Inpatient Utilization

The largest expense paid by an MCO is that of inpatient care. Every attempt is made to track and control the days that are paid for by the organization through proper case management and utilization management. The standard measure of inpatient utilization is bed days per 1,000 members, usually per one month/year. A *bed day* is the MCO equivalent of the hospital inpatient service day and is calculated in the same way. (See chapter 2.) The calculation result is rounded to a whole number for reporting purposes.

Some MCOs calculate bed days per 1,000 members separately for commercial, Medicare, and Medicaid members or bed days for adjusted member months, depending on the need to compare data with other organizations. The number of ED visits per 1,000 members also is a useful statistic kept by many MCOs.

For example, an MCO had the following statistics: 20,000 commercial members; 1,000 Medicaid members; 2,500 Medicare members; 1,200 ED visits for the month; 7,900 inpatient service days for the month (6,619 commercial inpatient service days, 356 Medicaid inpatient service days, and 925 Medicare inpatient service days); an HIM department staffing factor of .67; a commercial weighting factor of 1.0; a Medicaid weighting factor of 1.5; and a Medicare weighting factor of 2.5.

To find member months, add all the members together:

20,000	*Commercial*
1,000	*Medicaid*
+ 2.500	*Medicare*
23,500	*Total members for the month (member months)*

To find adjusted member months, multiply the members by the individual weighting factors, then add all the totals (this mix of members will use the resources of 27,750 commercial members for the month).

$$
\begin{array}{rcl}
20,000 \times 1.0 &=& 20,000 \\
1,000 \times 1.5 &=& 1,500 \\
2,500 \times 2.25 &=& +\ 6,250 \\
\hline
&& 27,750 \ \textit{adjusted member months}
\end{array}
$$

To find full-time employees (FTEs) for the HIM department per 1,000 members, divide the adjusted member months by 1,000. Then multiply this number by the number of HIM department staff members, as follows:

$$
\frac{27,750}{1,000} = 27.75 \qquad 27.75 \times .67 = 18.59 \ \textit{FTEs}
$$

To find *unadjusted* member months bed days per 1,000 members, divide total members for the month (member months) by 1,000. Then divide this number into total inpatient service days for the month, as follows:

$$
\frac{23,500}{1,000} = 23.50
$$

$$
\frac{7,900}{23.50} = 336.17 = \frac{336 \ \textit{unadjusted member months bed days}}{1,000}
$$

To find *adjusted* members months bed days per 1,000 members, divide total adjusted member months by 1,000. Then divide this number into total inpatient service days for the month, as follows:

$$
\frac{27,750}{1,000} = 27.75
$$

$$
\frac{7,900}{27.75} = 284.68 = \frac{285 \ \textit{adjusted member months bed days}}{1,000}
$$

To find commercial bed days per 1,000 members, divide the number of commercial members by 1,000. Then divide this number into commercial inpatient service days for the month, as follows:

$$
\frac{20,000}{1,000} = 20
$$

$$
\frac{6,619}{20} = 330.95 = \frac{331 \ \text{commercial bed days}}{1,000}
$$

To find Medicaid bed days per 1,000 members, divide the number of Medicaid members by 1,000. Then divide this number into Medicaid inpatient service days for the month, as follows:

$$\frac{1,000}{1,000} = 1$$

$$\frac{356}{1} = \frac{356 \; Medicaid \; bed \; days}{1,000}$$

To find Medicare bed days per 1,000 members, divide the number of Medicare members by 1,000. Then divide this number into Medicare inpatient service days for the month, as follows:

$$\frac{2,500}{1,000} = 2.5$$

$$\frac{925}{2.5} = \frac{370 \; Medicare \; bed \; days}{1,000}$$

To find the ED visits per 1,000 members, divide total members for the month (member months) by 1,000. Then divide this number into the number of ED visits for the month, as follows:

$$\frac{23,500}{1,000} = 23.5$$

$$\frac{1,220}{23.5} = 51.91 = \frac{52 \; emergency \; department \; visits}{1,000}$$

Exercise 10.1

1. How is resource allocation determined in most managed care organizations?

    a. Per member per month
    b. Medicare patients
    c. Medicaid patients
    d. Bed days

2. What is the MCO's largest expense?

    a. Laboratory tests
    b. X-ray exams
    c. ED visits
    d. Inpatient care

Ambulatory Care Facilities

Most ambulatory care statistics are maintained through the facility's finance or accounting department rather than its HIM department. Often the statistics are generated from the organization's practice management system or, in a smaller facility, its billing system. Commonly maintained statistics include:

- *Patient encounters per month:* Each time a patient receives services at the facility, the encounter is counted. The services may take place in the physician's office (appointment) or in laboratory, radiology, or other departments. Each encounter may generate multiple services (e.g., in one laboratory encounter, the patient may have blood tests, chemistry tests, and urine testing). Normally, encounters are reported by both provider and department.

- *RVUs (relative value units):* The RVU system, RBRVS (resource-based relative value system), was developed in the late 1980s as a structure for physician reimbursement through a prospective payment system (PPS). An RVU is assigned to each *CPT-4* code and based on a combination of three values: physician work, practice expense (overhead), and malpractice expense. Today, RVUs are used to establish fees for services and to track physician productivity. Physician compensation formulas generally incorporate the number of times each procedure/service was performed times the RVU for that procedure. These values are added together and then multiplied by some preestablished amount to arrive at physician income for the period.

- *Diagnosis and procedure frequency:* Ongoing diagnosis and procedure indices generally are not maintained in ambulatory care. When needed, a report is generated for a specific *ICD-9* or *CPT-4* code or a range of codes.

- *Tests:* Departments such as laboratory and radiology maintain statistics on the number of tests performed, based on *CPT-4* codes.

Long-Term Care Facilities

Many of the statistical formulas discussed in previous chapters are applicable to the long-term care (LTC) setting. Common statistics such as number of admissions, number of discharges, average monthly census, percentage of occupancy, and ALOS are important.

Figure 10.1 shows an example of a simplistic summary form that would assist the LTC facility in collecting and documenting some basic statistics. Figure 10.2 shows a statistical report for a long-term care facility.

However, as with other nontraditional settings, LTC statistics may vary from traditional acute care statistics. One example is a statistical report based on a skilled nursing facility (SNF) PPS. The Balanced Budget Act of 1997 mandated implementation of a per diem PPS for SNFs covering all costs related to the services furnished to beneficiaries under Part A of the Medicare program. Per diem payments for each admission are case-mix adjusted using a resident classification system (Resource Utilization Groups III, or RUGs) based on data from resident assessments (Minimum Data Set 2.0) and relative weights developed from staff time data.

Figure 10.1.	**Summary Report, YTD**											
1998	**Jan**	**Feb**	**Mar**	**Apr**	**May**	**Jun**	**Jul**	**Aug**	**Sep**	**Oct**	**Nov**	**Dec**
# of Admissions												
# of Discharges												
Average Monthly Census												
% of Occupancy												
Aver LOS (LT Unit)												
Aver LOS (ST Unit)												

Figure 10.2. **Long-term Care Statistical Report**

STATISTICAL REPORT

Month of: _____

Number of Admissions _____
Number of Evening Admissions _____

Number of Weekend Admissions _____

Source of Admissions:
    Home _____
    Hospital #1 _____
    Hospital #2 _____
    Other LTC _____

Common primary diagnoses:
    Neoplasm _____
    Infectious Disease _____
    Endocrine, Nutritional, Metabolic,
    Immunity _____
    Blood/Blood Forming organs _____
    Mental Disorders _____
    Nervous System and Sense Organs _____
    Circulatory System _____
    Respiratory System _____
    Digestive System _____
    Genitourinary _____
    Skin and Subcutaneous Tissue _____
    Musculoskeletal/Connective Tissue _____
    Congenital Anomalies _____
    S/S and ill defined conditions _____
    Injury and Poisoning _____

Average Daily Census for month _____
% of Occupancy for month _____

Average Case Mix for month: _____
Ave. Case Mix per primary pay source:
    Medical Assistance _____
    Medicare Part A _____
    Private Pay _____
    Managed Care _____

Number of Discharges: _____
Destination of Discharges:

    Death _____
    Other LTC _____
    Assisted Living _____
    Home _____
    Hospital _____
    AMA _____

Average LOS (LT Units): _____
Average LOS (ST Unit): _____

Number of Hospitalizations: _____
Reason(s) for Hospitalizations: _____
_____
_____

Number of Hosp. Returns: _____
Number of Evening Returns: _____
Number of Weekend Returns: _____

Number of Inquiries: _____
Source of Inquiries:
    Previous Resident _____
    Current Resident _____
    Hospital #1 _____
    Hospital #2 _____

Number of Residents per primary pay source:
    Medical Assistance _____
    Medicare A _____
    Private Pay _____
    HMO/Managed Care _____

Exercise 10.2

Below is an actual report taken from a Medicare study. Review the report and validate the numbers in bold and the percentages.

Staff Time Measure Study—Combined 1995 & 1997 Medicare Pop.

RUG III Categories & Subcategories	04/03/1998	Medicare MEDPAR Days Analysis Population	STM Percent of Pop.	95–97 STM Study Pop.
ADL INDEX		**28,336,126**		**3933**
REHABILITATION			Within Category	**1332**
ULTRA HIGH		**4,147,880**		343
RUC	16–18	544,183	**13.1%**	45
RUB	9–15	2,612,076	**63.0%**	216
RUA	4–8	991,621	**23.9%**	82
VERY HIGH		**2,793,310**		253
RVC	16–18	408,508	**14.6%**	37
RVB	9–15	1,402,175	**50.2%**	127
RVA	4–8	982,627	**35.2%**	89
HIGH		**4,410,117**		235
RHC	13–18	1,538,849	**34.9%**	82
RHB	8–12	2,101,843	**47.7%**	112
RHA	4–7	769,425	**17.4%**	41
MEDIUM		**10,599,033**		416
RMC	15–18	3,133,849	**29.6%**	123
RMB	8–14	5,528,823	**52.2%**	217
RMA	4–7	1,936,362	**18.3%**	76
LOW		**6,385,786**		85
RLB	14–18	1,953,299	**30.6%**	26
RLA	4–13	4,432,487	**69.4%**	59

Adapted from: *Federal Register*, 5/12/98, Table 2.C., page 26262–63

Behavioral Health Settings

As in other nontraditional settings, behavioral (mental) health statistics may vary from traditional acute care statistics. Common statistics such as LOS and age group are important. However, patients also may be categorized by diagnosis (such as schizophrenia), physical or mental state, GAF (global assessment of functioning) scale, or types of treatment and medications they are receiving.

In general, all behavioral health facilities use the GAF scale to report the patient's overall level of functioning: psychological, social, and occupational. The level of functioning is reported as a number between 1 and 100, with 100 representing the highest level.

One instrument used for substance-related diagnoses is the American Society of Addiction Medicine (ASAM) Patient Placement Criteria (PPC) for the treatment of substance-related disorders. The ASAM published a second edition of the *PPC (ASAM PPC-2)*, which contains the most widely used and comprehensive national guidelines for placement, continued stay, and discharge of patients with alcohol and other drug problems.

Exercise 10.3

The following table is an actual report from XYZ Mental Health Facility that calculates the percentage of improved level of functioning in comparison to the number of clients terminated. Review the report and then complete the worksheet that follows it.

XYZ Mental Health Facility
Level of functioning for clients who completed treatment
Month of September, 1999

Program	# Clients terminated per program	# with improved GAF score	# with same GAF score	# with lower GAF score	% improved level of functioning
Counseling	17	16	1	0	94%
Psychiatric Services 390, 392	4	3	1	0	75%
Emergency Services	1	1	0	0	100%
CIS	10	5	4	1	50%
CES	7	0	4	3	0%
Children's Outpatient	1	1	0	0	100%
BRIGGS	2	2	0	0	100%
CLP–CSP	3	0	3	0	0%
Older Adult Svcs Non-CSP	1	0	1	0	0%
Older Adult Scvs CSP	2	0	0	2	0%
Parent Aide	1	0	0	1	0%
Substance Abuse 310 + 311	4	3	1	0	75%
Day Tx 309	1	1	0	0	100%
Dual Diagnosis	2	0	0	2	0%
Totals	**56**	**32**	**15**	**9**	**57%**

Exercise 10.3 *(Continued)*

ABC Mental Health Facility
Level of functioning for clients who completed treatment
Month of October, 1999

Program	# Clients terminated per program	# with improved GAF score	# with same GAF score	# with lower GAF score	% improved level of functioning
Counseling	16	12	3	1	
Psychiatric Services 390, 392	1	0	0	1	
Emergency Services	0	0	0	0	
CIS	5	3	1	1	
CES	6	2	3	1	
Children's Outpatient	0	0	0	0	
BRIGGS	1	1	0	0	
CLP–CSP	0	0	0	0	
Older Adult Svcs Non-CSP	2	2	0	0	
Older Adult Scvs CSP	1	0	0	1	
MTT	2	0	1	1	
Project Reach	2	2	0	0	
Substance Abuse 310 + 311 + 314	6	5	1	0	
Day Tx 308	1	1	0	0	
Dual Diagnosis	2	0	1	1	
Totals	**45**	**28**	**10**	**7**	

Chapter 11
Measures of Variation

Objectives

At the conclusion of this chapter, you should be able to:

- Define and differentiate between range, variance, and standard deviation
- Calculate range, variance, and standard deviation.

Variability

In addition to measures of central tendency (discussed in chapter 1) in describing a distribution of numbers, it is important to provide information on the measure of spread, or variability (Hennekens and Buring 1987). The mean gives a measure of central tendency of a list of numbers but tells nothing about the spread of the numbers in the list. For example, review the following three groups:

Group A	3	5	6	3	3
Group B	4	4	4	4	4
Group C	10	1	0	0	9

Each of these groups has a mean of 4 ($^{20}/_5$), and yet it is clear that the amount of dispersion of variation within the groups is different. In addition to a measure of central tendency, another type of measure, called a *measure of variation,* is needed that describes how much the numbers vary. A measure of variation emphasizes differences (Lial and Miller 1979). *Variability* actually refers to the difference between each score and every other score, or the spread of the scores (Welkowitz, Ewen, and Cohen 1976).

Range

One simple descriptive measure of variation is range (Welkowitz, Ewen, and Cohen 1976). *Range* is the difference between the largest and smallest values in a frequency distribution. In reviewing the three groups in the previous section on variability, the largest number in group A is 6 and the smallest is 3, a difference of 3. In group B the difference is 0, and in group C the difference is 10. Therefore, the range for group A is 3, for group B the range is 0, and for group C the range is 10 (Lial and Miller 1979).

Range has the advantage of being easy to compute, and it can be useful as a *rough* measure of variability (Lial and Miller 1979). It is the simplest, order-based measure of spread, but it is far from optimal as a measure of variability for two reasons. First, as the sample size increases, the range also tends to increase. Second, because only two values (the most extreme values) are used in the calculation of range, it may give a misleading impression of true variability of the data (Hennekens and Buring 1987). Range is considered a nonresistant measure of spread. Thus, a preferable measure of variability would include the distribution of all the values, not just those at the extremes. More informative measures of variation are variance and standard deviation.

Exercise 11.1

Fourteen patients have the following lengths of stay: 2, 3, 3, 1, 4, 18, 3, 2, 1, 5, 4, 3, 6, 1. What is the range of this distribution of numbers?

Variance

As previously stated, variability actually refers to the difference between each score and every other score. For example, if there are 100 scores, you would have to compute the difference between the first score and each of the 99 other scores, and then compute the difference between the second score and each of the 98 remaining scores, and so on. There would be 4,950 differences in all. A more feasible approach, which serves the purpose equally well, is to define the differences or deviations of a single score in terms of how far it is from the average or the mean (Welkowitz, Ewen, and Cohen 1976).

Variance is the sum of squared deviations of individual values from the mean divided by the sample size reduced by one (Huffman 1994). It provides a summary of the dispersion of individual observations around the mean.

The formula for calculating variance is:

$$s^2 = \sum \frac{(x - \bar{x})^2}{n - 1}$$

where

s^2 = sample variance

$\sum$ = sum

x = value of a measure or observation

$\bar{x}$ = mean

n = number of values or observations

According to this formula, the variance is the average of the squared deviations from the mean. The more the values in a distribution are unequal, the greater the variance and standard deviation. In group B cited previously, the variance equals 0 because all the values are the same. Measures of variation equal zero when there is no variation. In the formula, variance is symbolized by using s^2. The symbol $\sum$ is used to denote the sum, $\bar{x}$ is the mean, and n is used to indicate the sample size. The term $n - 1$ is used in the denominator instead of n to adjust for the fact that the mean of the sample is used as an estimate of the mean of the underlying population. If the data are available from the entire population and not just a sample, $n - 1$ can be replaced by n (Hennekens and Buring 1987).

To calculate the variance using the previous data, a sample of fourteen patients has the following lengths of stay: 2, 3, 3, 1, 4, 18, 3, 2, 1, 5, 4, 3, 6, 1. In the next computation, x is the actual LOS per patient. The mean $\bar{x}$ LOS is calculated as follows:

$$\frac{56}{14} = 4 \; days$$

The order of the operations is to subtract the mean from each score, square each result, sum, and divide (Welkowitz, Ewen, and Cohen 1976).

The variance is computed as follows:

$$s^2 = \frac{240}{(14-1)} = \frac{240}{13} = 18.46$$

Patient	Length of Stay (x)	$(x - \bar{x})$	$(x - \bar{x})^2$
1	2	−2	4
2	3	−1	1
3	3	−1	1
4	1	−3	9
5	4	0	0
6	18	14	196
7	3	−1	1
8	2	−2	4
9	1	−3	9
10	5	1	1
11	4	0	0
12	3	−1	1
13	6	2	4
14	1	−3	9
Total Number of Patients **14**	**56**	**0**	**240**

The sum of the deviations from the mean is always equal to zero. Therefore, by squaring the differences from the mean, the negative and positive deviations do not cancel each other out. When squared, negative as well as positive values become positive (Lial and Miller 1979).

In this example, the size of the variance is influenced by the one LOS of 18 days. Removal of this value would result in a more homogeneous data set. The more the values in a distribution are unequal, the greater the variance and standard deviation.

In this chapter, use of the term *variance* refers to statistical variance, not budget variance. *Budget variance* is the difference between planned budgeted revenues and expenditures and actual revenues and expenditures for a given period.

Standard Deviation

Standard deviation (SD) is the square root of the variance. Because SD is the square root of the variance, it can be more easily interpreted as a measure of variation. In a normal distribution, one SD in both directions from the mean contains 68.3 percent of all values. Two SDs in both directions from the mean contain 95.5 percent of all values. Three SDs in both directions from the mean contain 99.7 percent of all observations. If the SD is small, there is less dispersion around the mean. If the SD is large, there is greater dispersion around the mean (SEER Program 1994).

The formula for calculating standard deviation is:

$$SD = \sqrt{\sum \frac{(x - \bar{x})^2}{(n - 1)}}$$

Continuing with the previous LOS example, the mean is 4 and the variance is 18.46. Thus, the SD is 4.3 (the square root of 18.46 = 4.29). This means that ±1 SD contains values ranging from 20.3 to 8.3; ± 2 SD includes values ranging fromm 24.6 to 12.6; and ±3 SD includes all values ranging from 28.9 to 16.9. Figure 11.1 shows a graph of standard deviation.

In evaluating the LOS data, we can conclude that 13 out of 14 (92.9%) length of stays fell within ±1 SD from the mean. The remaining value, 18, falls outside the ± 3 SD from the mean and thus is called an outlier.

Normal Distribution

The concept of normal distribution is one of the most important frequency distributions in statistics. In appearance, it is a symmetrical bell-shaped curve. Measurable characteristics tend to follow certain patterns. For instance, the frequency distribution of variables such as blood pressure, pulse rate, height, and serum cholesterol tend to take the shape of a normal distribution with little deviation from the average.

Normal distribution means that if the variable on every person in the population were measured, the frequency distribution would display a normal pattern, with most of the

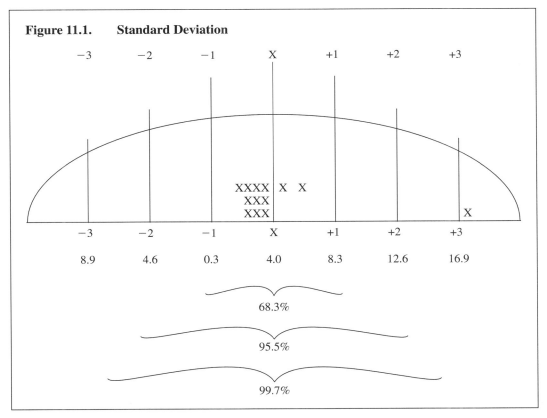

Figure 11.1.   Standard Deviation

(Huffman 1994)

measurements near the center of the frequency. It also would be possible to completely describe the population, with respect to variable, by calculating the mean, variance, and SD of the values (SEER Program 1994).

It should be noted that the distribution above is not a normal distribution. As stated earlier, in a normal distribution, one SD in both directions from the mean contains 68.3 percent of all values. In this data set, approximately 93 percent of the scores fall between ±1 SD from the mean. Visual inspection of the data reveals a fairly homogeneous data set despite the large SD. This emphasizes the importance of visual inspection of the data set when making decisions based on statistical calculations.

Test on Measures of Variation

The table below shows the lengths of stay for a sample of 11 discharged patients. Using the data in the table, calculate the mean, range, variance, and standard deviation for this set of values. Remember that:

$$s^2 = \sum \frac{(x - \bar{x})^2}{(n - 1)}$$

Patient	Length of Stay (x)	(x − x̄)	(x − x̄)²
1	1		
2	3		
3	5		
4	3		
5	2		
6	29		
7	3		
8	4		
9	2		
10	1		
11	2		
Total Number of Patients	**11**	**55**	**0**

Calculate the following:

1. Mean

2. Range

3. Variance

4. Standard deviation

5. What value is affecting the mean and standard deviation of this distribution?

6. Does the mean adequately represent this distribution? If not, what would be a better measure of central tendency for this data set?

Test Validation Exercise

The following actual report from a cancer registry shows the SDs of weights for twenty males with adenocarcinoma of the rectum. Validate the calculations used in the report.

Weights of Males with Adenocarcinoma of Rectum

Patient	Weight, lbs (x)	$(x - \bar{x})$	$(x - \bar{x})^2$
1	142	−30	900
2	148	−24	576
3	151	−21	441
4	155	−17	289
5	155	−17	289
6	158	−14	196
7	164	−8	64
8	165	−7	49
9	170	−2	4
10	173	1	1
11	175	3	9
12	175	3	9
13	175	3	9
14	183	11	121
15	185	13	169
16	186	14	196
17	189	17	289
18	193	21	441
19	198	26	676
20	200	28	784
Total Number of Patients **20**	**3,440**	**0**	**5,512**

*Standard deviation = 17.0; $s^2 = \dfrac{5,512}{19} = 290.1$; mean = 172; and $n - 1 = 19$

Chapter 12
Data Presentation

Objectives

At the conclusion of this chapter, you should be able to:

- Discuss categorical data: nominal (dichotomous), ordinal, interval, and ratio
- Differentiate between numerical data: discrete data and continuous data
- Describe and differentiate between tables and graphs
- Create tables and graphs to depict statistical information

Types of Data

Up to this point, you have calculated various sets of data. However, a set of data may not necessarily provide an examiner (such as an administrator, physician, or HIM professional) with information that can be easily interpreted (Lial and Miller 1979). *Descriptive statistics* deal with the collection, organization, and summarization of data. They provide an overview of the general features of a set of data. The statistics can assume a number of different forms, including tables and graphs. However, before discussing the various methods of displaying a set of data, you must first determine the type of data you have—categorical or numerical (Huffman 1994).

Categorical Data

There are four types of categorical data, or scales of measurement: nominal, ordinal, interval, and ratio (Pagano and Gauvreau 1993).

Nominal Data

Nominal data (dichotomous) are among the simplest types of data, where the values fall into unordered categories (Berthelsen and Nick 1995). Examples of nominal data include true/false, male/female, and diabetic/nondiabetic. Often numbers are used to represent categories (Pagano and Gauvreau 1993). For example, persons may be grouped according to blood type, where 1 represents type A; 2, type B; 3, type AB; and 4, type 0. The sequence of the values is not important. The numbers simply serve as labels for the different blood types.

Averages cannot be computed on nominal-level data. For example, an average blood type of 2.3 for a given population is meaningless. Instead of calculating the mean for nominal data, the proportion that falls into each category is reported.

Ordinal Data

Ordinal data are types of data where the values are in ordered categories or are ranked. These data are appropriate when the order of the categories is important, for example, to specify the degree of a patient's pain as minimal, moderate, severe, or unbearable (Berthelsen and Nick 1995). For example, head injuries may be classified according to level of severity, where 4 is fatal; 3, severe; 2, moderate; and 1, minor.

A natural order exists among the groupings, with the largest number representing the most serious level of injury. However, the order could be revised; there is no hard-and-fast rule. There is no reason why 1 could not represent the fatal injury and 4, the minor injury. In addition, the distance between a fatal and a severe injury may not necessarily be the same as the distance between a moderate and a minor injury. Intervals between ordered categories are not assumed to be equal (Pagano and Gauvreau 1993).

Ranked Data

Ranked data are types of ordinal data where the observations are first arranged from highest to lowest according to magnitude and then assigned numbers that correspond to each observation's place in the sequence. For example, it is possible to list all of the causes of death in the United States in 1999, along with the number of lives that each cause claimed. If the causes were ordered starting with the one that resulted in the greatest number of deaths and ending with the one that caused the fewest, and these were assigned consecutive integers, the data are said to be ranked. In ranked data, the relative position of the observation is considered and the magnitudes of the observations are disregarded (Pagano and Gauvreau 1993).

Table 12.1 shows an actual report listing the five leading causes of death in the United States in 1997. Note that cerebrovascular diseases would be ranked third whether they caused 539,576 or 109,030 deaths.

Table 12.1.	Five Leading Causes of Death in the United States, FY 1997	
Rank	**Cause of Death**	**Total Deaths**
1	Diseases of the heart	726,974
2	Malignant neoplasms	539, 577
3	Cerebrovascular diseases	159,791
4	Chronic obstructive pulmonary disease	109,029
5	Accidents and adverse effects	95,644

Reprinted with permission from *National Vital Statistics Reports,* Vol. 47, No. 19.

Interval Data

Interval data include units of equal size, such as intelligence quotient (IQ) results. *Ratio data* may be displayed by units of equal size placed on a scale starting with zero and thus can be manipulated mathematically, such as 0, 5, 10, 15, and 20 (Huffman 1994).

Numerical Data

Numerical data include discrete data and continuous data (Berthelsen and Nick 1995).

Discrete Data

Discrete data are finite numbers (SEER Program 1994). They can have only specified values. The number of children in a family is an example of discrete data. A family can have two or three children but cannot have 2.25 or 3.5 children. The numbers represent actual measurable quantities rather than labels. Other examples of discrete data include the number of motor vehicle accidents in Florida in 1992, the number of times a woman has given birth, the number of new cases of AIDS reported in the United States during a one-year period, and the number of beds available in a particular long-term care facility (Pagano and Gauvreau).

In discrete data, a natural order exists among the possible data values. In the example of the number of times a woman has given birth, a larger number indicates that she has had more children; the difference between one and two births is the same as the difference between four and five; and the number of births is restricted to whole numbers (a woman cannot give birth 2.3 times). For the most part, measurements on the nominal and ordinal scales are discrete.

Continuous Data

Continuous data represent measurable quantities but are not restricted to certain specified values (Pagano and Gauvreau 1993). Common examples of continuous data are blood pressure and serum cholesterol (Berthelsen and Nick 1995). Continuous data may have different or more precise values with successive refinements of the measuring scale. For example, height is continuous data. One could say that someone is approximately 6 feet tall, refine it to 5 feet 10 inches, and refine it still further to 5 feet 10½ inches. Other examples of continuous data include time and temperature (SEER Program 1994).

The only limiting factor for a continuous observation is the degree of accuracy with which it can be measured. For analysis, continuous data often are converted to a range that acts as a category. For example, age can be categorized in ranges (0–20, 21–40, and so on). Measurements on the interval and ratio scales are continuous (Pagano and Gauvreau 1993).

It is important to distinguish among the various types of data because different techniques are used to analyze them. The following section identifies the statistical techniques that are most appropriate for describing or summarizing each type of data discussed above (Pagano and Gauvreau 1993).

Data Display

Data display is critical to data analysis because it reveals patterns and behaviors. When preparing a statistical report, the user must define its objectives and scope. What information is needed? What information is available? Are the data collected routinely by the facility, or do additional data need to be collected?

If the purpose requires frequencies, percentages, or relationships among variables, the data may be presented in the form of a table or graph. Basically, statistical tables are used for summarizing data and graphs present data in a visual form. The question of whether to present data in the form of a table or a graph depends on the purpose of the report and its audience (SEER Program 1994).

There are a number of advantages to using tables, including:

- More information can be presented.

- Exact values can be read to retain precision.

- Supportive details can be provided.

- Less work and fewer costs are required in the preparation.

- Flexibility is maintained without distortion of data.

There also are many advantages to using graphs, including:

- They get the audience's attention.

- They are easy to understand.

- They bring out hidden facts.

- They vividly display trends or comparisons.

- A picture is worth a thousand words.

Tables

A table is the simplest means of summarizing a set of observations and can be used for all types of data (Pagano and Gauvreau 1993). It is an organized arrangement of data, usually into columns (reading down) and rows (reading across). The columns should be labeled. Many word-processing, spreadsheet, and database software programs offer assistance in the creation of tables. In table 12.2, variables are arranged in columns across the page that identify the individual patient name, age, clinical service, and length of stay (SEER Program 1994).

The essential components of a table include:

- *Title:* The title must explain as simply as possible what is contained in the table.

- *Stub heading:* The title or heading of the first column.

- *Column headings:* The headings or titles for the columns.

- *Stubs:* The categories (the left-hand column of a table).

- *Cells:* The information formed by intersecting columns and rows.

- *Source footnote:* The source for any data should be identified in a footnote.

Tables 12.3 and 12.4 below illustrate how these components should fall.

Table 12.2.   Analysis Showing Patients Discharged 12/1/99

Name	Age	Clinical Service	Length of Stay
Smith	5	Surgical	1
Valdez	22	Obstetrical	1
Chu	26	Obstetrical	2
MacDuff	18	Obstetrical	3
Johnson	10	Surgical	7
O'Brien	80	Surgical	8
Lewandowski	35	Surgical	11
Jones	52	Medical	15
Shultz	69	Medical	37
Martini	49	Medical	42

Table 12.3.   Sample Table Showing the Essential Components

	Title*		
Stub Heading	**Column Heading**	**Column Heading**	**Column Heading**
Stub	Cell	Cell	Cell
Stub	Cell	Cell	Cell
Stub	Cell	Cell	Cell

*Reprinted, with permission, from SEER Program, *Self-Instructional Manual for Cancer Registrars, Book 7* (Washington, D.C.: U.S. Department of Health and Human Services, 19940, p. 23.

Although these rules are important in the construction of tables, it is more important to use good judgment. Check the table to be sure that it is logical and self-explanatory. Are headings specific and understandable for every column and row? Do totals add up? Is it easy to read? Remember to present the data in a format to illustrate a specific idea.

Frequency Distribution Tables

The *frequency distribution table* is commonly used to evaluate data. For nominal and ordinal data, a frequency distribution table consists of a set of classes or categories, along with the numerical counts that correspond to each set. Table 12.5 is an actual report depicting the number of cigarettes smoked per adult in the United States (numerical count) in various years (classes or categories) (Pagano and Gauvreau 1993).

To display discrete or continuous data in the form of a frequency distribution table, the range of values of the observations must be broken down into a series of distinct groups that do not overlap. Summarizing the data involves setting up categories and counting the number of cases that fall into each category, thereby creating a frequency distribution.

Table 12.4.   Sample Table with Completed Components

Colon Cancer by Age and Sex at General Hospital*

	Age, years		
Sex	**<55**	**55–64**	**Total**
Male	30	42	72
Female	8	15	23
Total	**38**	**57**	**95**

---

*Cancer registry, 1985

Reprinted, with permission, from SEER Program, *Self-Instructional Manual for Cancer Registrars, Book 7* (Washington, D.C.: U.S. Department of Health and Human Services, 1994.

Table 12.5.   Actual Report Illustrating Frequency Distribution

Cigarette Consumption per Adult*
United States, 1960–1990*

Year	Number of Cigarettes Consumed
1960	4,171
1970	3,985
1980	3,851
1990	2,828

---

*Tobacco industry, 1992

Reprinted, with permission, from SEER Program, *Self-Instruction Manual for Cancer Registrars, Book 7* (Washington, D.C.: U.S. Department of Health and Human Services, 1994).

Following are some general rules for choosing the classes or categories into which the data are to be grouped and the range of each:

- As a general rule, do not use fewer than five or more than fifteen categories. The choice depends mostly on the number of values to be grouped.

- Categories should be well defined. Choose categories that cover the smallest and largest values and do not produce gaps between categories.

- The categories should be mutually exclusive where each observation is grouped into one—and only one—category. Avoid successive classes that overlap or have common values.

- Whenever feasible, categories should cover equal ranges of values (this rule does not apply to the open classes at the beginning and the end). The ranges should make sense in the context of the data (Huffman 1994).

Table 12.6 shows an example of a frequency distribution table.

Graphs

A *graph* proves the best medium for presenting data for quick visualization of relationships among various factors (SEER Program 1994). It is a pictorial representation of numerical data. Graphs should be designed to convey the general patterns in a set of data at a single glance (Pagano and Gauvreau 1993). They often supply a lesser degree of detail than tables. Data presented in a graph can be helpful in displaying statistics in a concise manner.

Graphs should be easy to read, simple in content, and correctly labeled. The presentation of data in the form of a graph is an excellent way to convey the message. Instead of using an entire statistical report in a presentation to a group (for example, medical staff or administration), you can create a graph to depict the data. Many computer software programs are available that convert data into graph form automatically and attractively.

Table 12.6   Example of a Frequency Distribution Table

Length of Stay for Patients Discharged at University Hospital, 12/1/95

Ages, in Years	# of Patients	Total Length of Stay
<16	2	12
16–30	3	6
31–50	2	53
51–64	1	15
65	2	45

The basic form of a graph is usually constructed by plotting numbers in relation to two axes (SEER Program 1994). The graph proceeds from left to right (horizontal axis) and bottom to top (vertical axis). The horizontal axis, referred to as the *x-axis,* notes independent variables such as scores, values, categories, or classes of data. The vertical axis, referred to as the *y-axis,* displays frequency (Huffman 1994). The vertical axis should always start with zero. The scale of values for the x-axis reads from the lowest value on the left to the highest on the right. The scale of values for the y-axis extends from the lowest value at the bottom of the graph to the highest at the top.

The essential components of a graph include:

- *Title:* The title must relate what the graph shows as simply as possible.

- *Legend or key:* When several variables are included on the same graph (that is, males or females), it is necessary to identify each by using a legend or key.

- *Scale captions:* Scale captions are placed on both axes to identify the values clearly.

- *Source footnote:* The exact reference to an outside source should be given.

On the one hand, selecting the most appropriate graph to accompany your data adds a great deal to the effectiveness of your presentation. However, an overabundance of graphs should be avoided. It is a good idea to produce several versions of a graph and then use the one that is most illuminating (SEER Program 1994).

Bar Graphs

Bar graphs, or bar charts, are used to display a frequency distribution for nominal or ordinal data (Pagano and Gauvreau 1993). The bar graph is the simplest form of graph (Huffman 1994). In it, the various categories of observations are presented along a horizontal axis. (See figure 12.1.) A vertical bar is drawn above each category so that its height represents the frequency of observations within that category (Pagano and Gauvreau 1993). Bar graphs are used to display categories of data that are not continuous (Huffman 1994). Data representing frequencies, proportions, or percentages of categories are often displayed using bar graphs. Bars are effective for displaying comparisons between groups such as the number or percent of cancer patients by race or stage of disease (SEER Program 1994).

Histograms

A *histogram* is the graph form used to display frequency distributions for continuous numerical data (interval or ratio data). Histograms are created by the representation of frequency groups (such as age ranges) on the horizontal axis. The vertical axis contains the frequency of observations. (See figure 12.2.) The first step in the construction of a histogram is to lay out the scales of the axes. The intersection of axes x and y should be zero. The vertical scale (y-axis) should begin at zero. If it does not begin with zero, visual comparisons among the intervals may be distorted. Vertical bars are then drawn to depict the frequency of each distribution or group (Pagano and Gauvreau 1993).

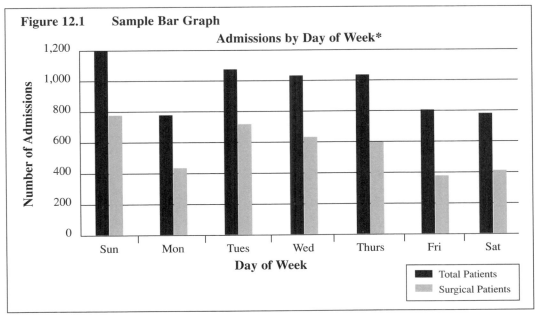

Figure 12.1   Sample Bar Graph

*Administrator's semiannual report from 1/1/99 to 6/30/99.

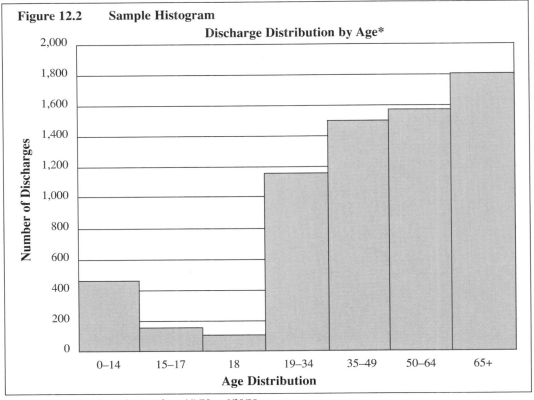

Figure 12.2   Sample Histogram

*Administrator's semiannual report from 1/1/99 to 6/30/99.

Following are a few rules to follow when creating a histogram:

- Establish between five and fifteen frequency groups.

- Form frequencies (y-axis) of equal dispersions to prevent distortion.

- Bars should be the same width and distributed evenly.

- Do not form overlapping frequency groups.

Line Graphs

A *line graph* is used to illustrate the relationship between continuous quantities (Pagano and Gauvreau 1993). This type of graph shows patterns or trends over some variable. Each point on the graph represents a pair of values. The line itself allows us to trace the change in the quantity of the y-axis that corresponds to a change along the x-axis. The x-axis has a single, corresponding measurement on the y-axis. The midpoints of the frequency groups are the points that connect the line.

The line graph is most often used to display time trends. (See figure 12.3.) The x-axis depicts the units of time from left to right, and the y-axis measures the values of the variable being shown. Consequently, the change in the quantity on the vertical axis can be traced over a specified period (SEER Program 1994).

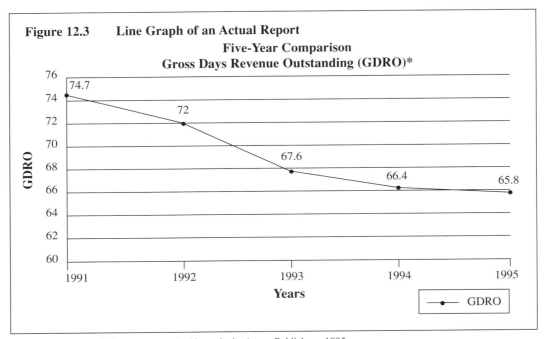

Figure 12.3   Line Graph of an Actual Report

Five-Year Comparison
Gross Days Revenue Outstanding (GDRO)*

*Prepared from hospital accounts receivable analysis, Aspen Publishers, 1995.

Pie Graphs

A *pie graph* is a method of displaying data as component parts of a whole. This type of graph pertains to one population, such as all patients discharged for a specific period of time. The pie graph, or pie chart, displays data by forming a circle that is divided into pie-shaped wedges. The wedges, or divisions, represent percentages of the total (100 percent). Some data may need to be converted into percentages. Pie graph wedges may be shaded or colored to help differentiate the sections. In addition, they can be cut out of the pie to help emphasize a percentage. Computer software programs are extremely useful when creating pie graphs (Huffman 1994; SEER Program 1994).

Figures 12.4 and 12.5 are pie graphs representing actual reports.

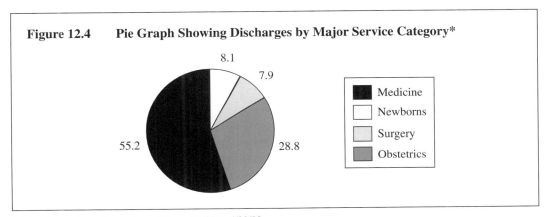

Figure 12.4   Pie Graph Showing Discharges by Major Service Category*

*Administrator's semiannual report from 1/1/99 to 6/30/99.

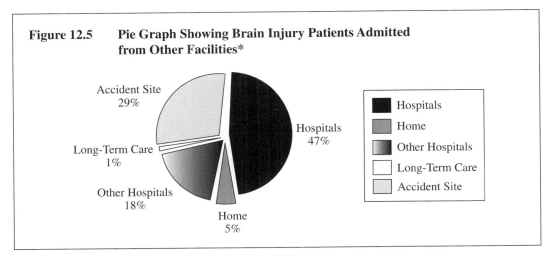

Figure 12.5   Pie Graph Showing Brain Injury Patients Admitted from Other Facilities*

*Rehabilitation hospital admissions report from 1/1/99 to 12/31/99.

Exercise 12.1

1. Indicate whether a table or a graph is the preferred method of presentation in the following situations:

    A. Distribution by site, sex, race, and time period of all cancers in your healthcare facility

    B. Survival trends over time by sex for lung cancer

    C. Display by stage of disease of prostate cancer to illustrate a presentation at a professional conference

    D. Detailed treatment distribution of breast cancer for a physician on the staff of your hospital

2. Indicate which of the following categories are mutually exclusive and clearly defined.

A	B	C
0–15	<10	0–10
15–30	10.1–20.0	11–20
30-45	20.1–30.1	21–39
45–60	30.1–40.0	40–50
60+	40.1–50.0	51+
50.1+		

Test on Data Presentation

Select the best answer to the following questions:

1. What is one of the simplest types of categorical data where the values fall into unordered categories?

    a. Ordinal
    b. Nominal
    c. Ratio
    d. Interval

2. What type of numerical data contains only a finite number of results?

    a. Continuous
    b. Discrete

3. In creating a frequency distribution table, which of the following statements is not a basic rule to follow:

   a. Choose classes that cover the smallest and largest values.
   b. Make certain that each item can go into only one class.
   c. As a general rule, use between ten and fifteen classes.
   d. Do not produce gaps between classes.

4. Line graphs can be used to illustrate the relationship between continuous quantities.

   a. True
   b. False

5. When creating histograms, which is a true statement?

   a. Form classes of equal width.
   b. Always form frequency groups that do not overlap.
   c. Establish between five and fifteen frequency groups.
   d. All of the above

6. Which graph displays vertical bars to depict frequency distributions for continuous data?

   a. Histogram
   b. Line graph
   c. Pie graph
   d. Frequency distribution table

7. Bar graphs are used to display comparisons between nominal data.
   a. True
   b. False

8. The wedges or divisions in a pie graph represent:
   a. Frequency groups
   b. Various data
   c. Percentages
   d. Classes

Assignment No. 3

Analyze the actual report on the next page and then prepare the following data displays. The data displays may be neatly hand drawn or created using a software program.

1. Create a histogram to display the distribution of total days by age.

2. Create a bar graph to display the admission by day of week for Medicare patients in comparison to the admission by day of week of total number of patients.

3. Create a pie graph to display the percentage of patients discharged by major service category.

4. Create a table for length of stay distribution.

Administrator's Semiannual Reference Report

ALL PATIENTS INCLUDING ONE-DAY STAYS (SEPARATE)

———————————— ADMISSIONS ———————————————————— DISCHARGES ————————

	TOTAL PTS.	% OF PTS.	AVG. LOS	SURG. PTS.	AVG. PRE-OP	ONE-DAY STAYS	TOTAL PTS.	% OF PTS.	AVG. LOS	ONE-DAY STAYS
SUNDAY	1,187	17.9	6.7	774	1.7	146	809	12.1	8.1	46
MONDAY	755	11.3	7.3	426	2.8	124	576	8.7	6.2	144
TUESDAY	1,085	16.3	7.5	689	2.6	135	934	14.0	7.2	115
WEDNESDAY	1,035	15.5	7.1	622	3.5	141	934	14.0	7.7	147
THURSDAY	1,024	15.3	6.3	597	2.6	139	955	14.3	7.0	132
FRIDAY	808	12.1	8.0	359	3.9	145	965	14.5	7.7	141
SATURDAY	773	11.6	9.1	417	3.0	39	1,490	22.4	6.6	144

— LENGTH OF STAY DISTRIBUTION —   ———————— SUMMARY BY MAJOR SERVICE CATEGORY ————————

	PATIENTS	% CASES		PTS.	% PTS.	DAYS	% DAYS	ALOS
SAME DAY	114	1.7	MEDICINE	2,005	30.0	21,052	30.6	10.4
1 DAY	755	11.3	SURGERY	1,401	21.0	7,845	11.4	5.5
2–4 DAYS	1,343	20.1	GYNECOLOGY	631	9.4	6,057	8.8	9.5
5–7 DAYS	1,555	23.3	OBSTETRICS	530	7.9	2,703	3.9	5.1
8–14 DAYS	1,469	22.0	NEWBORN	520	7.8	2,600	3.7	5.0
15–42 DAYS	1,217	81.3	PEDIATRICS	450	6.7	4,140	6.0	9.2
43+ DAYS	210	3.1	PSYCHIATRY	518	7.7	8,537	12.4	16.4
			OTHER	608	9.1	15,798	22.9	25.9

———————————— ADMISSION BY DAY OF THE WEEK BY PAYMENT STATUS ————————————

	SELF	BLUE CR	COMMERC	GOV'T	FREE	W.COMP.	U.M.W.	M-CAID	M-CARE	F.E.P.	TIT.V	HMO	OTHER
SUNDAY	31	413	188		2			41	273				2
MONDAY	19	300	103		11			46	280				1
TUESDAY	21	400	206	1	9			45	345				2
WEDNESDAY	20	503	240	2	22			35	223				3
THURSDAY	30	365	154		8			24	199				1
FRIDAY	28	402	179					42	294				
SATURDAY	30	509	246	1	6			55	301				2
TOTAL PTS.	179	2,892	1,316	4	58			288	1,915				11
% OF PTS.	2.6	43.4	19.7	0.6	0.8			4.3	28.7				0.0
TOTAL DAYS	1,109	26,895	16,818	36	609			2,670	20,491				104
% OF DAYS	1.6	39.1	24.4	0.0	0.8			3.8	29.8				0.0
AVG. LOS	6.1	9.2	12.7	9	10.5			9.2	10.7				9.4

———————————— SUMMARY BY AGE ————————————

	TOTAL PTS.	% OF PTS.	TOTAL DAYS	% DAYS	ALOS
0–14	429	6.4	1,749	2.5	4.1
15–17	140	2.1	420	.6	3.0
18	89	1.3	397	.6	4.5
19–34	1,144	17.2	9,746	14.2	8.5
35–49	1,488	22.3	14,647	21.3	9.8
50–64	1,570	23.6	18,101	26.3	11.5
65+	1,803	27.1	23,672	34.4	13.1
TOTAL	**6,663**		**68,732**		**10.3**

Chapter 13
Computerization of Statistics

Objectives

At the conclusion of this chapter, you should be able to:

- Verify computerized statistical reports for accuracy
- Recalculate statistics for greater specificity
- Generate computerized statistical reports

Verification of Reports

Many statistical reports in healthcare settings are computer generated. As previously discussed, the preparation of statistics involves the collection, analysis, interpretation, and presentation of facts as numbers. Because HIM practitioners possess a broad range of knowledge about healthcare facilities, they are in the best position not only to collect and prepare data, but also to analyze and interpret them.

However, a computer can only calculate statistics from the data that are entered. Standardization of terminology, data elements, and formulas from sources such as appendix B (*Glossary of Healthcare Services and Statistical Terms*) will result in data that are more reliable and useful.

When a computerized statistical report is received, the HIM practitioner should examine it carefully. For example, he or she should verify the total number of discharges listed in a report from discharged abstracts and compare it to the total number of discharges according to the census data. Do the totals match? If not, was one of the discharges not abstracted? Moreover, computerized statistical reports often give only whole numbers. Thus, the HIM practitioner may need to calculate certain statistics (for example, death rates) and carry them out to the second decimal place to make the information more valuable to administration or the medical staff. Tables or graphs can be created to display a portion of a computerized statistical report. (See chapter 12.)

Computerized Discharge Reports

Figure 13.1 shows an actual report titled "Discharge Analysis" that indicates the average length of stay (ALOS) of total patients is 7.3 days. To verify this information, use your knowledge of ALOS and recalculate. The calculation is:

$$\frac{4{,}713}{650} = 7.25 = 7.3$$

Another verification can be done by adding the percentages given for the day-of-the-week admissions and the day-of-the-week discharges to make certain they add up to 100 percent. In the computerized statistical report above, they do add up to 100 percent (13 + 13 + 18 + 15 + 17 + 14 + 10 = 100 and 7 + 12 + 14 + 19 + 14 + 19 + 15 = 100). These data could be presented in the form of a pie graph. (See chapter 12.)

Computerized Financial Statistical Reports

A computer also can be used to compile various financial statistical reports. An actual computerized financial report titled "Most Frequent DRGs by Financial Class" is shown in figure 13.2. Note that the ALOS is rounded to a whole number. For example, for heart failure and shock, the ALOS is 6 days. If you recalculate the ALOS and carry it to the second decimal place, it is 5.80.

$$\frac{1{,}252}{216} = 5.796$$

Computerized Readmission Rate Report

Figure 13.3 shows a computerized readmission rate report. This type of report delineates inpatients by medical service and calculates each medical service's readmission rate.

Case-Mix Index Report

Figure 13.4 shows an actual report titled "Case Mix Index report." This report depicts the facility's case-mix index for all financial classes for the month and then the fiscal year to date. It also extrapolates the case-mix index for Medicare-only patients.

Exercise 13.1

1. The report in figure 13.1 gives the gross death rate (hospital death rate) as 01 percent. Recalculate this rate and carry your answer to the second decimal place.

2. Using the report in figure 13.1, recalculate the gross autopsy rate carrying out the answer to the second decimal place.

3. Using the report in figure 13.1, what is the ALOS of Medicare patients? of Blue Cross patients?

4. Looking at the financial report in figure 13.2, what is the ALOS for the total number of patients?

5. Using the report shown in figure 13.2, which diagnosis-related group (DRG) has the greatest ALOS?

6. Analyze the report in figure 13.3 and recalculate the readmission rates to verify their accuracy. Also, calculate the overall readmission rate.

7. Analyze the report in figure 13.4 and recalculate the rates to verify their accuracy. How many Medicare patients were discharged fiscal year to date? What month end was this report calculated?

8. Review the actual report on page 124 for physician profile A. Recalculate the consultation rates to verify their accuracy. (Note that there is no information in this category for physicians 10125 and 15007.)

Use of Spreadsheets

Numerous statistical software packages are available for the creation of spreadsheets. Spreadsheets, or worksheets, allow you to enter text, numbers, and formulas to assist in calculations. A spreadsheet usually consists of columns that are lettered across the top of the document and rows that are numbered down the left side of the document. The intersections of columns and rows form cells, which are the basic units for storing data.

Each software package varies slightly in technique. Most packages perform basic arithmetic functions as well as many of the statistical calculations discussed in this book. Various add-in features allow for data sorting, formatting for printing data, and even graphical interface. Most software packages contain a help section, as well as a tutorial to assist the novice. The best way to gain proficiency with any software package is to "just do it" and practice, practice, practice.

Figure 13.1. **Actual Computerized Discharge Analysis Report**

* * * YOUR UTILIZATION PROGRAM * * *

SERVICE	TOTAL			AGE ANALYSIS						PATIENTS OPERATED	EMERGENCY ADMISSIONS	CONSULTATION	
				0-13 YEARS		14-64 YEARS		65 AND OVER				NO. OF PATIENTS	NUMBER RECEIVED
	PATIENTS	DAYS	AVG. STAY	PAT.	DAYS	PAT.	DAYS	PAT.	DAYS				
1	2	3	4	5	6	7	8	9	10	11	12	13	14
MEDICINE	204	1880	9.2	1	2	161	1300	42	578	170	3	128	209
CARDIOLOGY	60	626	10.4			43	436	17	190	44	1	17	21
ENDOCRINOLOGY	2	23	11.5			2	23			2		2	3
GASTROENTEROL	13	99	7.6			13	99			13		6	11
ONCOLOGY	17	178	10.5			10	112	7	66	16		8	15
PULMONARY MED	4	40	10.0			4	40			4		1	1
PSYCHIATRY	3	17	5.7			2	14	1	3	1		2	6
OB-LIVE BIR	26	114	4.4			26	114			25		2	3
OB-NOT DELIV	9	23	2.6			9	23			4			
OB-ABOR FETUS	15	26	1.7			15	26			15		1	1
GYNECOLOGY	33	125	3.8			33	125			31		5	11
NEWBORN	25	130	5.2	25	130					6			
PED MED	47	265	5.6	44	217	3	48			30	1	8	11
PED SURG	5	11	2.2	4	9	1	2			5		2	2
PED ORTHO	5	27	5.4	2	10	3	17			5		4	5
PED RHINOLARYN	2	3	1.5	1	1	1	2			1		1	1
PED OPHTH	1	2	2.0	1	2					1		1	1
PED UROL	1	1	1.0	1	1					1			
SURGERY	35	222	6.3	1	2	31	190	3	30	34	2	13	18
CV SURG	7	74	10.6			6	72	1	2	7		4	5
ORTHOPEDICS	77	551	7.2	1	11	73	506	3	34	74	1	51	78
PLAS SURG	4	8	2.0			4	8			4		1	1
PROCTOLOGY	1	5	5.0			1	5			1			
ORAL SURG-ADU	3	6	2.0			3	6			3			
UROLOGY	23	172	7.5			18	131	5	41	22		12	16
OPHTHALMOLOGY	5	18	3.6			3	9	2	9	5		2	2
RHINOLARYNG	5	17	3.4	1	1	3	13	1	3	5		1	1
ADULT T & A	2	4	2.0			2	4			2			
PED T & A	1	1	1.0	1	1					1			
PODIATRY	15	45	3.0			14	41	1	4	15		5	6
TOTALS INC / NB	650		7.3	83		484		83		547		277	
		4713			387		3366		960		8		428
LESS NEWBORNS	25	130											
TOTALS EXC / NB	625	4583											

TOTAL CASES	AVG. STAY	TRANSFERRED TO					LENGTH OF STAY DISTRIBUTION			
		OTHER HOSP.	SNF		HOME CARE		1 – 3 DAYS	4 – 14 DAYS	15 – 30 DAYS	OVER 30 DAYS
			UNDER 64	65 AND OVER	UNDER 64	65 AND OVER				
625	7.3	8	1	7			28%	62%	10%	%

% OF PATIENTS OPERATED	% OF EMERG ADM.	% OF PATIENTS W/ CONS	AVG. # OF CONS	TRANSFER RATE		
				TO OTHER HOSP.	TO SNF	TO HOME CARE
84%	01%	43%	2	1.2%	1.2%	

HOSP # XXXX   JAN 1999   PAGE 1

ALIVE STATUS 15	AMA 16	TRANSFER 17	DEATHS				COMMERCIAL		BLUE CROSS		MEDICAID		MEDICARE	
			EXP NO AUT 18	EXP AUT 19	COR. CASE NO AUT 20	AUT 21	PAT. 22	DAYS 23	PAT. 24	DAYS 25	PAT. 26	DAYS 27	PAT. 28	DAYS 29
184	4	14	2				39	323	72	625	28	172	53	700
56		2	1	1			9	60	20	235	5	43	24	273
2											1	9	1	14
13							3	20	7	54	1	11	2	14
14			3				4	38	4	44	2	30	7	66
4							3	33			1	7		
		3					1	5	1	9			1	3
26							2	14	7	34	2	52		
9							1	1	1	1	6	20		
15							2	4	9	14	2	5		
33							7	22	16	51	10	52		
25							2	11	6	33	13	55		
47							12	73	16	91	18	100		
5							2	3	3	8				
5							3	19	1	7				
2									2	3				
1									1	2				
1											1	1		
33			1	1			11	57	19	107			4	38
6		1					2	22	2	21			3	31
76		1					29	233	20	161	8	21	4	46
4									3	7	1	1		
1							1	5						
3									3	6				
23							5	27	10	73	2	19	5	41
5									3	9			2	9
5							2	3	2	11			1	3
2									2	4				
1							1	1						
15							4	11	7	23	3	7	1	4
616	4	21	7	2			145	985	237	1633	114	605	108	1242

DEATHS						OTHER PAYMENT STATUS							
GROSS DEATH RATE	NET DEATH RATE	GROSS AUT. RATE	NET AUT. RATE	COR CASES	POST-OP	SELF-PAY		WORK-COMP		FREE OTHER – GOV		UMW	
						PAT	DAYS	PAT	DAYS	PAT	DAYS	PAT	DAYS
01%	01%	22%	22%			26	124	18	107	1	9		

DAY OF WEEK OF ADMISSION							DAY OF WEEK OF DISCHARGE						
SUN	MON	TUES	WED	THURS	FRI	SAT	SUN	MON	TUES	WED	THURS	FRI	SAT
13%	13%	18%	15%	17%	14%	10%	07%	12%	14%	19%	14%	19%	15%

Figure 13.2. **Actual Computerized Financial Report**

MOST FREQUENT DRGS BY FINANCIAL CLASS (R1-19)

For Discharges from 01/01/99 to 12/31/99

F/C incl: MC   P/T excl: H,D,I,T,U

FINANCIAL CLASS	DRG CODE	DRG DESCRIPTION	# OF PATS.	PAT DAYS	ALOS	TOTAL CHARGES
MEDICARE	127	HEART FAILURE & SHOCK	216	1252	6	2,125,018.00
MEDICARE	14	SPECIFIC CEREBROVASCULAR DISORDERS EXCEPT TIA	141	1009	7	1,798,011.89
MEDICARE	209	MAJOR JOINT AND LIMB REATTACHMENT PROCEDURES	136	926	7	2,601,090.62
MEDICARE	89	SIMPLE PNEUMONIA & PLEURISY AGE >17 WITH C.C.	117	807	7	1,271,445.45
MEDICARE	88	CHRONIC OBSTRUCTIVE PULMONARY DISEASE	98	579	6	920,071.41
MEDICARE	174	G.I. HEMORRHAGE WITH C.C.	94	487	5	964,597.03
MEDICARE	79	RESPIRATORY INFECTIONS & INFLAMMATIONS AGE >17 WITH C.C.	88	905	10	1,656,856.52
MEDICARE	148	MAJOR SMALL & LARGE BOWEL PROCEDURE WITH C.C.	88	1092	12	2,493,260.52
MEDICARE	182	ESOPHAGITIS, GASTROENT & MISC DIGES DISORDERS, AGE >17 WITH CC	86	324	4	560,025.93
MEDICARE	210	HIP & FEMUR PROCEDURES EXCEPT MAJOR JOINT AGE >17 WITH C.C.	81	617	8	1,329,055.73
MEDICARE	138	CARDIAC ARRHYTHMIA & CONDUCTION DISORDERS WITH C.C.	71	290	4	506,803.44
MEDICARE	140	ANGINA PECTORIS	70	234	3	466,286.80
MEDICARE	416	SEPTICEMIA AGE >17	69	619	9	1,209,069.85
MEDICARE	296	NUTRITIONAL & MISC METABOLIC DISORDERS AGE >17 WITH C.C.	63	366	6	532,230.77
MEDICARE	124	CIRCULATORY DISORDERS EXCEPT AMI, W CARD CATH & COMPLEX DIAG	56	248	4	687,146.08
MEDICARE	15	TRANSIENT ISCHEMIC ATTACK AND PRECEREBRAL OCCLUSIONS	52	158	3	336,667.38
MEDICARE	121	CIRCULATORY DISORDERS WITH AMI & C.V. COMP DISCH ALIVE	51	328	6	790,417.76
MEDICARE	320	KIDNEY & URINARY TRACT INFECTIONS AGE >17 WITH C.C.	47	240	5	367,789.93
MEDICARE	87	PULMONARY EDEMA & RESPIRATORY FAILURE	43	369	9	707,485.01
MEDICARE	410	CHEMOTHERAPY	41	85	2	198,692.68

Figure 13.2. *(Continued)*

FINANCIAL CLASS	DRG CODE	DRG DESCRIPTION	# OF PATS.	PAT DAYS	ALOS	TOTAL CHARGES
MEDICARE	180	G.I. OBSTRUCTION WITH C.C.	39	235	6	386,509.40
MEDICARE	116	OTH PERM CARDIAC PACEMAKER IMPLANT OR AICD LEAD / GENERATOR	33	146	4	592,506.88
MEDICARE	188	OTHER DIGESTIVE SYSTEM DIAGNOSES AGE >17 WITH C.C.	33	218	7	427,499.12
MEDICARE	144	OTHER CIRCULATORY SYSTEM DIAGNOSES WITH C.C.	31	189	6	447,102.64
MEDICARE	475	RESPIRATORY SYSTEM DIAG WITH VENTILATOR SUPPORT	31	387	12	1,215,601.28
MEDICARE	404	LYMPHOMA & NON-ACUTE LEUKEMIA W/O C.C.	1	4	4	4,011.41
MEDICARE	406	MYELOPROLIF DISORD OR POORLY DIFF NEOPLASM W MAJ O.R. PROC W C.C.	1	23	23	45,480.70
MEDICARE	424	O.R. PROCEDURES WITH PRINCIPAL DIAGNOSIS OF MENTAL ILLNESS	1	20	20	26,289.88
MEDICARE	428	DISORDERS OF PERSONALITY & IMPULSE CONTROL	1	19	19	15,508.06
MEDICARE	442	OTHER O.R. PROCEDURES FOR INJURIES WITH C.C.	1	14	14	35,775.10
MEDICARE	444	MULTIPLE TRAUMA AGE >17 WITH C.C.	1	4	4	5,560.30
MEDICARE	447	ALLERGIC REACTIONS AGE >17	1	5	5	10,687.30
MEDICARE	454	OTHER INJURIES, POISONING & TOXIC EFFECT DIAG WITH C.C.	1	2	2	6,522.35
MEDICARE	455	OTHER INJURIES, POISONING & TOXIC EFFECT DIAG W/O C.C.	1	2	2	3,161.58
MEDICARE	460	NON-EXTENSIVE BURNS W/O O.R. PROCEDURE	1	3	3	3,302.98
MEDICARE	463	SIGNS & SYMPTOMS WITH C.C.	1	6	6	9,279.07
MEDICARE	479	OTHER VASCULAR PROCEDURES W/O C.C.	1	2	2	23,031.87
MEDICARE	485	HIP, FEMUR, AND LIMB REATTACH PROC FOR MULTI SIGN TRAUMA	1	7	7	21,149.70
MEDICARE	486	OTHER O.R. PROCEDURES FOR MULTIPLE SIGNIFICANT TRAUMA	1	5	5	14,882.29
MEDICARE	490	HIV W/ OR W/O OTHER RELATED CONDITO	1	4	4	7,104.30
MEDICARE	492	CHEMOTHERAPY WITH ACUTE LEUKEMIA AS SECONDARY DIAGNOSIS	1	10	10	28,618.33
		TOTALS	3360	21833	6	45,462,381.17
		LOCATION	3360	21833	6	45,462,381.17

Figure 13.3.   Computerized Readmission Rate Report

XXXXXXXXXXXX Hospital
Readmission Rate
For Month End   10/98

Case Type	Number of Readmits	Number of Cases	Readmit Rate
I	188	2046	9.18

Readmission Rate by Service
For Month End   10/98

Case Type	Medical Service	Number of Readmits	Number of Cases	Readmit Rate
I	ABS		3	.00
I	ABT		1	.00
I	ALL		1	.00
I	CRD	10	277	3.61
I	CVS	10	84	11.90
I	DLC	5	70	7.14
I	DLN		16	.00
I	DLR		53	.00
I	END		2	.00
I	FPR	5	75	6.66
I	GI	5	27	18.51
I	GYN	1	68	1.47
I	INF	1	8	12.50
I	MED	59	511	11.54
I	MON	26	67	38.80
I	NB	1	129	.77
I	NEU	1	4	25.00
I	NIC		21	.00
I	NIN		1	.00
I	NPH	42	162	25.92
I	NRS		25	.00
I	OB	3	80	3.75
I	ONR		1	.00
I	OPH		1	.00
I	ORS	2	14	14.28

Figure 13.3.   *(Continued)*

Case Type	Medical Service	Number of Readmits	Number of Cases	Readmit Rate
I	ORT	4	84	4.76
I	OTO		11	.00
I	PED	1	55	1.81
I	PPA	1	2	50.00
I	PUL		4	.00
I	RON	2	2	100.00
I	RPL		11	.00
I	SUR	4	71	5.63
I	THS	3	37	8.10
I	URO	1	42	2.38
I	VSS	1	26	3.84
I			2046	

Figure 13.4.   **Computerized Case-Mix Index Report**

XXXXXXXXXXXX Hospital
Case Mix Index Report – All Financial Classes
For Fiscal Year to Date   99

Total Weight	Number of Cases	Case Mix Index
6831.0912	3230	2.1148

Case Mix Index Report—Medicare Only
For Fiscal Year to date   99

Total Weight	Number of Cases	Case Mix Index
2915.2882	1367	2.1326

Case Mix Index Report—All Financial Classes
For Month End   10/98

Total Weight	Number of Cases	Case Mix Index
3396.8017	1626	2.0890

Case Mix Index Report—Medicare Only
For Month End   10/98

Total Weight	Number of Cases	Case Mix Index
1364.1506	658	2.0731

Physician Profile A

ATTEN. PHYS.	CASES	TOTAL SURG. CASES	DAYS	EMER. CL PTS.	AVG. LOS	PRE-OP LOS
01000	202	18	1,111	69	5.5	3.1
01005	182	21	1,911	49	10.5	5.5
01006	259	42	2,719	88	10.3	4.5
01009	242	29	2,250	79	9.3	3.8
04000	53	6	509	9	9.6	4.0
10125	1	1	2		2.0	1.0
15000	3	3	31	1	10.3	1.0
15002	76	10	737	19	9.7	4.6
15006	188	18	1,354	64	7.2	5.6
15007	2		18	2	9.0	
15008	95	5	751	32	7.9	4.0
TOTAL	1,303	153	11,393	412	8.7	3.7

Assignment No. 4

1. In chapter 4, turn to the table used in exercise 4.2 (see page 39). Using the list of 10 patients by name, age, clinical service, and LOS, create a computerized spreadsheet to calculate the ALOS.

2. In chapter 8, review the example from Huffman's tenth edition of *Health Information Management* in the section on adjusted hospital autopsy rate (see page 68). Create a simple spreadsheet to calculate the adjusted hospital autopsy rate.

3. Using the table below from the section on calculating inpatient service days in chapter 2, create a spreadsheet to calculate service days for June 2 and 3.

Day	12:00 census A/C	Nb	adm A/C	b	trf in	total A/C	Nb	dis A/C	Nb dis	trf out	11:59 census A/C	Nb	a/d	serv days A/C	Nb
6/1	48	2	2	1	1	51	3	1	2	1	49	1	1	50	1
6/2	49	1	3	1	2	54	2	4	1	2	48	1	1		
6/3			1	1	1			3	0	1			0		

		DEATHS					PTS. RECEIVING CONSULTS		
TOT.	% OF DTHS	POST- OP	W48 ADM	AUT CAS	COR CAS	TOT PTS.	CONS REC'D	AVG. CONS.	CONS RATE
12	5.9	1		1		72	104	1.4	36%
14	7.7		2	1		93	146	1.6	51%
15	5.8	2	2	1		122	175	1.4	47%
18	7.4	1	3	1	1	117	162	1.4	48%
4	7.5		1			30	43	1.4	57%
						1	1	1.0	33%
4	5.3		1	1		55	93	1.7	72%
7	3.7	1	1	1	1	77	103	1.3	41%
4	4.2			2		55	76	1.4	58%
78	6.0	5	10	8	2	622	903	1.4	48%

References and Bibliography

Abdelhak, Mervat. 1996. *Health Information: Management of a Strategic Resource*. Philadelphia: W. B. Saunders Company.

American Society for Testing and Materials. *1999 Annual Book of ASTM Standards*; *Volume 14.0 Health Informatics; Computerized Systems and Chemical and Material Information*; *Standard Guide for Content and Structure of the Computer-Based Patient Record E 1384*. West Conshohocken, Pa.: ASTM.

Austrin, Michael. 1999. *Managed Health Care Simplified: A Glossary of Terms*. Albany, N.Y.: Delmar Thomson Learning.

Babbie, E. 1983. *The Practice of Social Research*. 3rd edition. Belmont, Calif.: Wadsworth Publishing.

Bertheisen, C. L., and T. G. Nick. 1995. Statistical inference in health information management. *Journal of American Health Information Management Association* (July–August).

Bertheisen, C. L., and T. G. Nick. 1995. Application of statistical inference techniques in health information management. *Journal of American Health Information Management Association* (October).

Downing, D., and J. Clark. 1989. *Statistics the Easy Way*. 2nd edition. New York City: Barron's.

Fletcher, Donna M. 1999. Reimbursement at your fingertips—A glossary of terms. *Journal of American Health Information Management Association* 70:8 (September), p. 60–72.

Hanken, Mary Alice. 1994. *Glossary of Healthcare Terms*. Chicago: American Health Information Management Association.

Health Care Finanacing Administration. 1998. *Outcome and Assessment Information Set (OASIS-B1)* (November). Washington, D.C.: U.S. Department of Health and Human Services.

Hennekens, C. H., and J. E. Buring. 1987. *Epidemiology in Medicine*. Boston: Little Brown & Co.

Huffman, E. K. 1994. *Health Information Management*. 10th edition. Berwyn, Ill.: Physician's Record Company.

Joint Commission on Accreditation of Healthcare Organizations. 1998. *Lexikon: Dictionary of Healthcare Terms, Organizations and Acronyms*. 2nd edition. Oakbrook, Ill: JCAHO.

Lial, M., and C. Miller. 1979. *Mathematics with Applications in the Management, Natural, and Social Science*. Glenview, Ill.: Scott Foresman & Co.

Medicode. 1999. *Coders' Desk Reference*. Salt Lake City: Medicode.

Miller, Susan. 1996. *Documentation and Information Management in Home Care and Hospice Programs*. Chicago: American Health Information Management Association.

National Center for Health Statistics. 1997. Ten leading causes of death in the U.S. *National Vital Statistics Reports*, Vol. 47, No. 19. Washington, D.C.; NCHS

National Committee on Vital and Health Statistics. 1996. *Core Health Data Elements* (August). Washington, D.C.: NCVHS

Pagano, M., and K. Gauvreau. 1993. *Principles of Biostatistics*. Belmont, Calif.: Duxbury Press.

Rognehaugh, Richard. 1998. *The Managed Health Care Dictionary*. 2nd edition. Gaithersburg, Md.: Aspen Publishing.

SEER Program. 1994. *Self-Instructional Manual for Cancer Registrars, Book 7: Statistics and Epidemiology for Cancer Registries*. National Institutes of Health, Public Health Service. Washington, D.C.: U.S. Department of Health and Human Services.

Snipes, K. P., C. L. Perkins, W. E. Wright, and J. L. Young. 1994. *Cancer Incidence and Mortality by Race/Ethnicity in California, 1988–1991*. Sacramento, Calif.; California Department of Health Services, Cancer Surveillance Section (May).

United Nations Statistics Division. 1997. *World Population Prospects: The 1996 Revision,* supplemented by *Population and Vital Statistics Report:* Data available as of 1 July 1997. Washington D.C.; United Nations Statistics Division.

U.S. Public Health Service. 1988. Standard terminology for reporting of reproductive health statistics in the United States. *Public Health Reports* 103:5, 464–71 (September–October). Washington D.C.; U.S. Public Health Service.

Welkowitz, J. R., B. Ewen, and J. Cohen. 1976. *Introductory Statistics for the Behavioral Science*. 2nd edition. New York City: Academic Press.

Review Exercises

Review Exercise 1 (Assignment No. 5)

Using the statistics provided, complete the fourteen calculations below. Use a separate sheet of paper to write your answers. Carry answers to the hundredth (two decimal places) and round to the tenth (one decimal place).

The following figures are for a hospital with 217 beds and 30 bassinets for the month of December:

Admissions
Adults and children 689
Newborns. 139

Inpatient Service Days
Adults and children 4,815
Newborns. 451

Deaths
Adults and children
    Under 48 hours. 5
    48 hours and over. 10
Newborns
    Under 48 hours. 3
    48 hours and over. 0
Outside hospital 2
Fetal deaths
    Under 20 weeks 4
    20 weeks and over 2
Postoperative 1
On surgical service. 4

Surgery
Total surgical operations. 422
Surgical patients discharged 195

Miscellaneous

Coroner's cases not autopsied. 2
Patients receiving consultation 152
Deliveries. 138
Cesarean sections. 8
Hospital infections 13
Postoperative infections 3

Discharges and Deaths

Adults and children 647
Newborns. 128

Discharge Days

Adults and children 4,268
Newborns. 362

Autopsies

Adults and children
    Under 48 hours. 1
    48 hours and over. 9
Newborns
    Under 48 hours. 3
    48 hours and over. 0
Outside hospital 2
Fetal deaths
    Under 20 weeks 0
    20 weeks and over 2

Calculate the following:

1. Average daily census

2. Bed occupancy ratio

3. Average length of stay (excluding newborns)

4. Death rate

5. Postoperative death rate

6. Neonatal mortality (death) rate

7. Fetal death rate

8. Average daily newborn census

9. Adjusted hospital autopsy rate

10. Net autopsy rate

11. Postoperative infection rate

12. Consultation rate

13. Cesarean section rate

14. Hospital infection rate

Review Exercise No. 2 (Assignment No. 6)

Using the statistics provided, complete the thirteen calculations below. Use a separate sheet of paper to write your answers. Carry answers to the hundredth (two decimal places) and round to the tenth (one decimal place).

The following figures are December statistics for a hospital with 200 beds from December 1–20; 250 beds from December 21–31; and 20 bassinets for the entire month. The beginning census on December 1 at 12 A.M. (including newborns) was 201.

Admissions
Adults & children. 610
Newborns (livebirths). 112

Inpatient Service Days
Adults & children 6,352
Newborns. 395

Deaths
Adults & children
   Under 48 hours. 3
   48 hours and over. 18
Newborns
   Under 48 hours. 1
   48 hours and over. 2
Fetal deaths
   Under 20 weeks 4
   20 weeks and over 2
Postoperative 1
On surgical service. 4

Surgery
Total surgical operations. 280
Surgical patients discharged 60

Miscellaneous
Coroner's cases not autopsied 2
Patients receiving consultation 126
Deliveries. 98

Discharges and Deaths
Adults & children. 570
Newborns. 90

Discharge Days
Adults & children 6,652
Newborns. 489

Autopsies
Adults & Children
   Under 48 hours. 2
   48 hours and over. 8

Newborns

    Under 48 hours. 1
    48 hours and over. 0
On stillborn 1
On former patients by hospital pathologist 3

Calculate the following:

1. Consultation rate

2. Fetal death rate

3. Adjusted hospital autopsy rate

4. Net autopsy rate

5. Death rate

6. Postoperative death rate

7. Ending census on December 31 at 11:59 P.M.

8. Average daily census

9. Average length of stay

10. Bed occupancy ratio

11. Neonatal (mortality) death rate

12. Bassinet occupancy ratio

13. Average daily newborn census

Review Exercise No. 3 (Assignment No. 7)

Complete the following exercises:

1. The midpoint of the distribution of values is:

    a. Mean
    b. Median
    c. Mode
    d. Range

2. The number of inpatients present at the census-taking time each day plus any inpatients who were both admitted and discharged after the census-taking time the previous day is the:

    a. Census
    b. Daily inpatient census
    c. Total inpatient service days
    d. Percentage of occupancy

3. The medical unit of a hospital has 50 beds. During August, the unit provided 1,420 inpatient days of service. What was the average daily census for that unit in August?

    a. 28
    b. 45
    c. 46
    d. 47

4. An alternative term for *bed count* is:

    a. Bed complement
    b. Bed capacity
    c. Both a and b
    d. None of the above

5. Which statement concerning LOS is not true?

    a. The day of discharge is counted.
    b. The day of admission is counted.
    c. Subtract the date of admission from the date of discharge when the patient is admitted and discharged within the same month.
    d. Adding days is necessary to calculate LOS when it extends one or more months.

6. The death of a liveborn infant within the first 27 days, 23 hours, and 59 minutes from the moment of birth is the definition of a:

    a. Postneonatal death
    b. Stillbirth
    c. Infant death
    d. Neonatal death

7. Which of the following statements is true concerning hospital death rate?

    a. Patients who are dead on arrival (DOA) are included.
    b. Death is a type of discharge.
    c. Fetal deaths are included.
    d. Patients who die in the ED are included.

8. The main difference between net autopsy rate and adjusted hospital autopsy rate is:

    a. Fetal deaths are not counted in hospital autopsy rates.
    b. Hospital autopsy rates include only those patients whose bodies are available for autopsy.
    c. Net autopsy rate considers only inpatient deaths.
    d. Legal cases are sometimes excluded from deaths when computing net autopsy rate.

9. Which graph depicts sections of the whole?

    a. Histogram
    b. Line graph
    c. Pie graph
    d. Frequency distribution table

10. In creating a frequency distribution table, which of the following statements is not a basic rule to follow?

    a. Choose classes that cover the smallest and largest values.
    b. Make certain each item can go into only one class.
    c. As a general rule, use between 10 to 15 classes.
    d. Do not produce gaps between classes.

Appendix A
Formulas

Adjusted Hospital Autopsy Rate Formula:

$$\frac{\textit{Total hospital autopsies} \times 100}{\textit{Total number of deaths of patients whose bodies are available for hospital autopsy}}$$

Average Daily Census for a Care Unit Formula:

$$\frac{\textit{Total inpatient service days for the unit for the period}}{\textit{Total number of days in the period}}$$

Average Daily Census Formula:

$$\frac{\textit{Total inpatient service days for a period (excluding newborns)}}{\textit{Total number of days in the period}}$$

Average Daily Newborn Census Formula:

$$\frac{\textit{Total newborn inpatient service days for a period}}{\textit{Total number of days in the period}}$$

Average Length of Stay Formula:

$$\frac{\textit{Total length of stay (discharge days)}}{\textit{Total discharges (including deaths)}}$$

Average Newborn Length of Stay Formula:

$$\frac{\textit{Total newborn discharge days}}{\textit{Total newborn discharges (including deaths)}}$$

Bed Occupancy Ratio Formula:

$$\frac{Total\ inpatient\ service\ days\ in\ a\ period \times 100}{Total\ bed\ count\ days\ in\ the\ period\ (bed\ count \times number\ of\ days\ in\ the\ period)}$$

Bed Turnover Rate Direct Formula:

$$\frac{Number\ of\ discharges\ (including\ deaths)\ for\ a\ period}{Average\ bed\ count\ during\ the\ period}$$

Bed Turnover Rate Indirect Formula:

$$\frac{Occupancy\ rate \times number\ of\ days\ in\ a\ period}{Average\ length\ of\ stay}$$

Cancer Mortality Rate Formula:

$$\frac{Number\ of\ cancer\ deaths\ during\ a\ period \times 100,000}{Total\ number\ in\ population\ at\ risk}$$

Cesarean Section Rate Formula:

$$\frac{Total\ number\ of\ cesarean\ sections\ performed\ in\ a\ period \times 100}{Total\ number\ of\ deliveries\ in\ the\ period\ (including\ cesarean\ sections)}$$

Death Rate Formula:

$$\frac{Number\ of\ deaths\ of\ inpatients\ in\ a\ period \times 100}{Number\ of\ discharges\ (including\ deaths)\ in\ the\ period}$$

Fetal Death Rate Formula:

$$\frac{Total\ number\ of\ intermediate\ and/or\ late\ fetal\ deaths\ for\ a\ period \times 100}{Total\ number\ of\ live\ births + Intermediate\ and\ late\ fetal\ deaths\ for\ the\ period}$$

Gross Autopsy Rate Formula:

$$\frac{Total\ inpatient\ autopsies\ for\ a\ period \times 100}{Total\ inpatient\ deaths\ for\ the\ period}$$

Maternal Mortality Rate Formula:

$$\frac{Number\ of\ direct\ maternal\ deaths\ for\ a\ period \times 100}{Number\ of\ obstetrical\ discharges\ (including\ deaths)\ for\ the\ period}$$

Mean Formula:

$$\frac{\text{Total of all the values (sum)}}{\text{Number of the values involved}} = \bar{x}$$

Neonatal Mortality (Death) Rate Formula:

$$\frac{\text{Total number of newborn deaths for a period} \times 100}{\text{Total number of newborn infant discharges (including deaths) for the period}}$$

Net Autopsy Rate Formula:

$$\frac{\text{Total inpatient autopsies for a period} \times 100}{\text{Total inpatient deaths} - \text{Unautopsied coroners' or medical examiners' cases}}$$

Newborn Bassinet Occupancy Ratio Formula:

$$\frac{\text{Total newborn inpatient service days for a period} \times 100}{\text{Total newborn bassinet count} \times \text{Number of days in the period}}$$

Other Rates Formula:

$$\frac{\text{Number of times something occurred} \times 100}{\text{Number of times something could have occurred}}$$

Postoperative Infection Rate Formula:

$$\frac{\text{Number of infections in clean surgical cases for a period} \times 100}{\text{Number of surgical operations for the period}}$$

Standard Deviation (SD) Formula:

$$SD = \sqrt{\sum \left[\frac{(x - \bar{x})^2}{(n - 1)} \right]}$$

Variance Formula:

$$s^2 = \sqrt{\sum \left[\frac{(x - \bar{x})^2}{(n - 1)} \right]}$$

where

$s^2 = $ sample variance

$\sum = $ sum

$x = $ value of a measure or observation

$\bar{x} = $ mean

$n = $ number of values or observations

Vital Statistics Rates Formulas

Infant Mortality Rate Formula:

$$\frac{\textit{Number of infant deaths (neonatal and postneonatal) during a period} \times 1,000}{\textit{Number of live births during the period}}$$

Maternal Mortality Rate Formula:

$$\frac{\textit{Number of deaths attributed to maternal conditions during a period} \times 100,000}{\textit{Number of live births during the period}}$$

Neonatal Mortality Rate Formula:

$$\frac{\textit{Number of neonatal deaths during a period} \times 1,000}{\textit{Number of live births during the period}}$$

Postneonatal Mortality Rate Formula:

$$\frac{\textit{Number of postneonatal deaths during a period} \times 1,000}{\textit{Number of live births during the period}}$$

Appendix B
Glossary of Healthcare Services
and Statistical Terms
by Barbara Glondys, RHIA

AAAHC: *See* Accreditation Association for Ambulatory Health Care

Abortion: The expulsion or extraction of all (complete) or any part (incomplete) of the placenta or membranes, without an identifiable fetus or with a liveborn infant or a stillborn infant weighing less than 500 grams. In the absence of known weight, an estimated length of gestation of less than 20 completed weeks (139 days), calculated from the first day of the last normal menstrual period, may be used.

Accreditation: A determination by an accrediting body that an eligible organization, network, program, group, or individual complies with applicable standards.

Accreditation Association for Ambulatory Health Care (AAAHC): An accreditation authority for ambulatory healthcare entities. Originally the Joint Commission's ambulatory review function, the AAAHC became a separate organization in 1979. The association's services include the development of standards, performance measurement, consulting, and education. The AAAHC reviews care quality, QA, clinical records, environmental safety, governance, administration, and professional development.

Activities of daily living (ADL): The activities usually performed for oneself in the course of a normal day, such as eating, dressing, washing, combing hair, brushing teeth, and taking care of bodily functions. An ADL checklist is often used by providers to assess a patient prior to hospital discharge. If activities cannot be adequately performed, arrangements should be made with an outside agency (such as a visiting nurse service) or with family members to provide the necessary assistance.

Actual charge: A physician's actual fee for service at the time the insurance claim is submitted to the insurance company, government payer, or HMO.

Acute care: Short-term care. For inpatients, acute care indicates an average hospital stay of 30 days or less; for outpatients, acute care indicates care of short duration.

Adjunct diagnostic or therapeutic unit (ancillary unit): An organized unit of a hospital—other than an operating room, delivery room, or medical care unit—with facilities and personnel to aid physicians in the diagnosis and treatment of patients through the performance of diagnostic or therapeutic procedures.

Adjusted hospital autopsy rate: The proportion of hospital autopsies performed following the deaths of patients where the bodies of the deceased are available for autopsy.

ADL: *See* Activities of daily living

Admission date (inpatient): The year, month, and day of admission. An inpatient admission begins with a hospital's formal acceptance of a patient who is to receive healthcare practitioner or other services while receiving room, board, and continuous nursing services.

Admission type: Admissions are classified for UB-92 purposes into several types of inpatient admissions. These categories are:

> *Emergency:* The patient requires immediate medical intervention as a result of severe, life-threatening, or potentially disabling conditions. (Generally, the patient is admitted through the emergency department.)

> *Urgent:* The patient requires immediate attention for the care and treatment of a physical or mental disorder. (Generally, the patient is admitted to the first available and suitable accommodation.)

> *Elective:* The patient's condition permits adequate time to schedule the availability of a suitable accommodation.

> *Newborn:* A baby born within this facility.

Admitting diagnosis: A statement of the provisional condition given as the basis for admission to the hospital for study.

Adult day care: Daytime groups or individual service to persons outside their homes by an agency frequently used for the aging or the emotionally disturbed.

Advance directive: A legal, written document that specifies patient preferences regarding future healthcare or the person who is authorized to make medical decisions in the event the patient is not capable of communicating his preferences. The patient must be competent at the time the document is prepared and signed. Living wills and durable power of attorney are both considered advance directives.

Aftercare: The type of healthcare services that are sequentially provided after some period of hospitalization or rehabilitation, which are administered based on each patient's condition, with the objective of improving or restoring health to the degree that aftercare is no longer needed. Aftercare may include any or multiple continuum options under post-acute care.

Alias: A name added to, or substituted for, the proper name of a person; an assumed name.

ALOS: *See* Average length of stay

Ambulatory care/outpatient care: Preventive or corrective healthcare, or both, provided in a practitioner's office, clinic setting, or in a hospital on a nonresident basis (that is, not requiring overnight stay and not included in the census). While many inpatients may be ambulatory, the term ambulatory care usually implies that the patient has come to a location other than his or her home and has departed that same day. Ambulatory care includes non-medical healthcare sites (for example, acupuncture).

Ambulatory care organization/service: An organization or service, including individual providers, which offers preventive, diagnostic, therapeutic, and rehabilitative services to individuals not classified as inpatients or residents.

Ambulatory patient groups (APGs): Similar to DRGs (diagnosis related group), APGs are used to categorize ambulatory patients into case types to provide a pricing mechanism for outpatient services. Also called *ambulatory care groups* and *ambulatory visit groups*. In 2000, APGs were replaced with ambulatory payment classifications (APCs), authorized by the 1997 passing of the Balanced Budget Act.

Ambulatory payment classifications (APCs): A Medicare prospective payment system for hospital outpatient services, certain Part B services furnished to inpatients who have no Part A coverage, and partial hospitalization services furnished by community mental health centers. The Balanced Budget Act of 1997 authorized the Health Care Financing Administration to implement this prospective payment system for outpatient services, which became effective August 1, 2000.

Ambulatory surgery: A program for the performance of elective surgical procedures on patients who are classified as outpatients and typically are released from the surgery center on the day of surgery.

Ambulatory surgery center: A free-standing or hospital-based facility offering surgical procedures on patients who are admitted and discharged from the facility on the day of the surgery.

Ambulatory surgery organization/service: An organization or service that performs surgical procedures on patients who are classified as outpatients and typically released from the facility within several hours after surgery.

American Society for Testing and Materials (ASTM): An organization whose purpose is to establish standards of materials, products, systems, and services. Founded in 1898 and headquartered in Conshohocken, Pennsylvania, ASTM has developed 9,000 standard test methods and recommended practices now in use.

Ancillary services/professional service departments: Hospital diagnostic and/or therapeutic services provided to both outpatients and inpatients, excluding room and board.

Ancillary service visit: The appearance of an outpatient in a unit of a hospital or outpatient facility to receive service(s), test(s), or procedures. An ancillary service visit is ordinarily not counted as an encounter.

Ancillary unit: *See* Adjunct diagnostic or therapeutic unit

Anesthesia death rate: The ratio of deaths caused by anesthetic agents to the number of anesthetics administered during a specified period of time.

Anesthetic risk: The risk of harm caused by anesthetic agents. Any procedure that either requires or is regularly performed under general anesthesia carries anesthetic risk, as do procedures under local, regional, or other forms of anesthesia that induce sufficient functional impairment necessitating special precautions to protect the patient from harm.

APCs: *See* Ambulatory payment classifications

APGs: *See* Ambulatory patient groups

Assignment of benefits: The transfer of one's interest or policy benefits to another party, typically the payment of medical benefits directly to a provider of care. This circumstance generally requires either a contract between the health plan and the provider or a written release from the subscriber to the provider allowing the provider to bill the health plan.

ASTM: *See* American Society for Testing and Materials

Attending physician: The physician responsible for the care and treatment of a patient.

Attending physician identification (inpatient): The unique national identification number assigned to the clinician of record at discharge who is responsible for the discharge summary.

Autopsy rate: The proportion of deaths that are followed by the performance of an autopsy. It can include the gross, net, and adjusted autopsy rates.

Available for hospital autopsy: The following conditions must be met before a hospital autopsy can be performed:

- The body of a current or former hospital patient has been transported to the appropriate facility;

- necessary authorization has been secured from the relatives;

- the hospital pathologist has agreed to perform the autopsy;

- the autopsy report will be filed in the patient's hospital medical record and the hospital laboratory; and

- the tissue specimens will be filed in the hospital laboratory.

The hospital patients whose bodies after death are available for hospital autopsy include:

- Inpatients, unless the bodies are removed from the hospital by legal authorities (coroners, medical examiners, anatomical boards). However, in any such case, if the hospital pathologist or delegated physician of the medical staff performs an autopsy while acting as an agent for the coroner, the autopsy is included in the numerator and the death in the denominator.

- Other hospital patients (including hospital home care patients, outpatients, and previous hospital patients who have died elsewhere) whose bodies have been made available for the performance of hospital autopsies.

Average daily census: The average number of inpatients present each day for a specified period of time.

Average duration of hospitalization: *See* Average length of stay

Average length of stay (ALOS): The average length of stay of inpatients discharged during a specified period of time.

Average stay: *See* Average length of stay

Balance billing: The practice of a provider billing a patient for all charges not paid by the insurance plan because those charges are above the plan's usual, customary, and reasonable practice or may be considered medically unnecessary. Plans are increasingly prohibiting providers from balance billing except for allowed copays, coinsurance, and deductibles.

Balanced Budget Act of 1997 (BBA): Bipartisan budget legislation signed on August 5, 1997, which added new penalties against fraud. These new provisions include such penalties as permanent exclusion for those convicted of three health-related crimes on or after the date of enactment and mandated prospective payment systems for outpatient and home health services.

Bar chart/bar graph: A graph used to display a frequency distribution or nominal or ordinal data.

BBA: *See* Balanced Budget Act of 1997

Bed capacity: 1. *See* Bed count. 2. The number of beds that a facility has been designed and constructed to contain, rather than the actual number of beds set up and staffed for use.

Bed count/bed complement: The number of available facility inpatient beds, both occupied and vacant, on any given day.

Bed count day: A unit of measure denoting the presence of one inpatient bed (either occupied or vacant) set up and staffed for use in one 24-hour period.

Bed occupancy ratio: The proportion of beds occupied, defined as the ratio of inpatient service days to bed count days during a specified period of time.

Bed size: The total number of inpatient beds for which the facility is equipped and staffed for patient admissions.

Bed turnover rate: The number of times a bed, on the average, changes occupants during a specified period of time.

Behavioral healthcare: A broad array of mental health, chemical dependency, forensic, mental retardation, developmental disabilities, and cognitive rehabilitation services provided in settings such as acute, long-term, and ambulatory care.

Benefit levels: The degree to which a person is entitled to receive services based on his/her contract with a plan or insurer.

Birth weight: The weight of a neonate determined immediately after delivery or as soon thereafter as feasible. Weight should be expressed to the nearest gram.

Birth weight of newborn (inpatient): The specific birth weight of the newborn, recorded in grams.

Board certified: A designation given to a physician or other health professional who has passed an exam from a medical specialty board and is thereby certified to provide care within that specialty.

Boarder: An individual who receives lodging at a healthcare facility but is not a patient. A boarder may be a parent, caregiver, or other family member who wishes or needs to be near the patient.

Boarder baby: 1. A newborn who remains in the nursery following discharge because the mother is still hospitalized. 2. A premature infant who no longer needs intensive care but remains for observation.

Cafeteria Plan: A health plan that allows employees to "pick and choose" among two or more benefits. With this type of plan, an employer can provide employees with a choice of taxable or nontaxable benefits; employees are taxed only to the extent of the value of the taxable benefit chosen. Plan options may include accident or health insurance and dependent care assistance.

Calculation of inpatient service days: The measurement of the services received by all inpatients in one 24-hour period.

Calculation of transfers: The medical care unit shows transfers on and off the unit as subdivisions of patients admitted to and discharged from the unit.

Capitation: A reimbursement method in which healthcare providers receive a prepaid fixed fee for each person enrolled in a managed care setting. This fee is compensation for all health services provided to members during a specified period of time, regardless of how much or how often resources are used.

Care: The management of, responsibility for, or attention to the safety and well-being of another or other persons.

Care unit: An organizational entity of a healthcare facility. Healthcare facilities are organized both physically and functionally into units to provide care.

Case management: The ongoing review of cases by professionals to assure the most appropriate utilization of services.

Case manager: A medical professional (usually a nurse or social worker) who reviews cases to determine necessity of care and to advise providers on payer's utilization restrictions. The case manager certifies ongoing care.

Case mix: A method by which patients are grouped together based on a set of characteristics (such as resource consumption, diagnosis, or procedure).

Case mix index (CMI): A single number that compares the overall complexity of the hospital's Medicare patients to the complexity of the average of all hospitals.

Categorical data: Also called *scales of measurement,* there are four types of categorical data: nominal, ordinal, interval, and ratio.

CCU: *See* Coronary care unit

Census: The number of inpatients present in the healthcare facility at any given time.

Census Statistics: Statistics that examine the number of patients being treated at specific times, length of their stay, and number of times a bed changes occupants.

Certificate of need: A state-directed program that requires facilities to submit detailed plans and justifications for the purchase of new equipment, new building, or new service offerings that cost in excess of a certain amount. The state review committee determines whether the proposed service or structure is needed. If approved, a certificate to proceed is extended.

Certification: The procedure and action by which a duly authorized body evaluates and recognizes (certifies) an individual, institution, or educational program as meeting pre-determined requirements (such as standards). Certification differs from accreditation in that certification can be applied to individuals whereas accreditation is applied only to institutions or programs.

Cesarean section rate: The ratio of all cesarean sections to the total number of deliveries—including cesarean sections—during a specified period of time.

CHAMPUS: *See* Civilian Health and Medical Program of the Uniformed Services

Charge master/charge description master: A report that reflects the charge for each item that may be used in the treatment of a patient and the charge for most services (such as respiratory therapy treatments, physical therapy services, and laboratory tests).

Chief complaint: The presenting problem

Civilian Health and Medical Program of the Uniformed Services (CHAMPUS): A federal program providing supplementary civilian-sector hospital and medical services beyond that which is available in military treatment facilities to military dependents, retirees and their dependents, and certain others.

Claim: A bill for healthcare services submitted to a third-party payer for payment of benefits under a healthcare insurance plan.

Classification system: The grouping of related entities to produce necessary statistical information.

Clinic: An outpatient facility providing a limited range of healthcare services, and assuming overall healthcare responsibility for the patients.

Clinical service: A general term used to indicate a unit of medical staff responsibility (such as cardiology), a unit of inpatient beds (such as general medicine), or even a group of discharged patients with related diseases or treatment (such as orthopedic).

Clinic outpatient: An outpatient who is admitted to a clinical service of the clinic or hospital for diagnosis or treatment on an ambulatory basis. Hospitals and clinics may organize into units of medical or surgical specialties or subspecialties.

Clinic patient: A person admitted for diagnosis or treatment or follow-up on an ambulatory basis; the clinic assumes overall medical responsibility for the patient.

Clinic referral: *See* Source of admission

Closed panel: A health plan or medical/dental group practice whose beneficiaries are allowed to use only those specified facilities and physicians or dentists that accept the plan's or organization's conditions of membership and reimbursement.

CMI: *See* Case mix index

COBRA: *See* Consolidated Omnibus Budget Reconciliation Act of 1975

Coinsurance: A health insurance term indicating that the insured is responsible for a portion or percentage of the healthcare cost.

Comorbidity: A pre-existing condition that will, because of its presence with a specific principal diagnosis, cause an increase in the patient's length of stay by at least one day in 75 percent of the cases.

Complication: 1. An additional diagnosis that describes a condition arising after the beginning of hospital observation and treatment and modifying the course of the patient's illness or the medical care required. 2. A condition that arises during the hospital stay that prolongs the patient's length of stay by at least one day in 75% of the cases.

Comprehensive outpatient program: An outpatient program for the prevention, diagnosis, and treatment of any illness, defect, or condition that prevents the individual from functioning in an optimal manner.

Computer-based patient record (CPR): An electronic patient record that resides in a system specifically designed to support users by providing accessibility to complete and accurate data, alerts, reminders, clinical decision support systems, links to scientific knowledge, and other aids.

Concurrent conditions: Physical disorders present at the same time as the primary diagnosis that alter the course of the treatment required or lengthen the expected recovery time of the primary condition.

Conditions of Participation: *See* Medicare Conditions of Participation

Consolidated Omnibus Budget Reconciliation Act of 1975 (COBRA): A federal law requiring every hospital that participates in Medicare and has an emergency room to treat any patient in an emergency condition or active labor, whether or not covered by Medicare and regardless of ability to pay. COBRA also requires employers to provide continuation benefits to specified workers and families who have been terminated but previously had benefits.

Consultation: The response by one healthcare professional to another healthcare professional's request to provide recommendations and/or opinions regarding the care of a particular patient/resident. The consultation usually requires an examination of the patient/resident, review of the patient/resident's history and diagnostic data, and documentation of the feedback provided.

Continuing care retirement community: An organization established to provide housing and services, including healthcare, to people of retirement age.

Continuous data: Data that represent measurable quantities but are not restricted to certain specified values.

Coordination of benefits: The prevention of double payment for services when an enrollee has coverage from two or more sources.

Copayment: A type of cost-sharing in which the insured (subscriber) pays out of pocket a fixed amount for healthcare services.

COPs: *See* Medicare Conditions of Participation

Coronary care unit (CCU): A facility dedicated to patients suffering from heart attack, stroke, or other serious cardiopulmonary problems.

Correct coding initiative (CCI): A Medicare initiative designed to improve the accuracy of Part B claims processed by Medicare carriers. The CCI was first implemented in 1996 and includes 93,000 computer edits. These edits are designed to detect claims with codes for services that cannot or should not be performed together or for services that should be grouped together and paid as one item at a lower rate rather than billed separately.

Cost outliers: *See* outliers

Court/law enforcement referral: *See* source of admission

CPR: *See* Computer-based patient record

CPT-4: *See* Current Procedural Terminology

Current Procedural Terminolgy (CPT-4): A nomenclature, developed by the American Medical Association, that lists descriptive terms and identifying codes for reporting medical services and procedures performed by physicians.

Custodial care: Care that is not directed toward a cure or restoration to a previous state of health but includes medical or non-medical services provided to maintain a given level of health without skilled nursing care.

Daily census: The number of inpatients present at the census-taking time each day, plus any inpatients who were both admitted after the previous census-taking time and discharged before the next census-taking time.

Date of birth: The year, month, and day of birth. It is recommended that the year of birth be recorded in four digits to make the data element more reliable for the increasing number of patients 100 years and older.

Date of encounter (outpatient and physician services): The year, month, and day of an encounter, visit, or other healthcare encounter.

Date of procedure (inpatient): The year, month, and day of each significant procedure.

Date of service: The year, month, and day of healthcare service.

Day on leave of absence: A day occurring after admission and prior to the discharge of a hospital inpatient when the patient is not present at the census-taking hour because he or she is on leave of absence from the healthcare facility.

Days of stay: *See* Length of stay

Dead on arrival (DOA): The condition in which a patient arrives at a healthcare facility with no life processes and is pronounced dead by a physician.

Death rate: The proportion of inpatient hospitalizations that end in death.

Deductible: The amount of cost that the beneficiary must incur before the insurance plan will assume liability for remaining costs.

Deemed status: An official designation that a healthcare facility is in compliance with the Medicare *Conditions of Participation*. To receive deemed status, facilities must be accredited by the Joint Commission on Accreditation of Healthcare Organizations or the American Osteopathic Association.

Delivery: The procedure of delivering a liveborn infant or dead fetus (and placenta) by manual, instrumental, or surgical means.

Delivery room: A special operating room for obstetric delivery and infant resuscitation.

Dependent: An enrolled health plan member who has coverage tied to that of a sponsor. A dependent may be a spouse, an unmarried child, or a stepchild or legally adopted child of either the employee or the employee's spouse, whose primary domicile is with the employee.

Descriptive statistics: Statistics that deal with the collection, organization, and summarization of data. They describe characteristics of a population derived from a sample.

Developmental disability: A mental or physical limitation affecting major life activities, arising before adulthood, and usually lasting throughout life. Developmental disabilities can be grouped into four major categories: autism, cerebral palsy, epilepsy, and mental retardation.

Diagnoses: All diagnoses that affect the current hospital stay.

Diagnosis: A word or phrase used by a physician to identify a disease from which an individual patient suffers or a condition for which the patient needs, seeks, or receives medical care.

Diagnosis chiefly responsible for services provided (outpatient): The diagnosis, condition, problem, or the reason for encounter/visit that is chiefly responsible for the services provided. If a definitive diagnosis has not been established at the end of the visit/encounter, the condition should be recorded to the highest documented level of specificity (such as symptoms, signs, abnormal test results, or other reason for visit).

Diagnosis related groups (DRGs): A Method of case mix adopted by the federal government and some other payers as a prospective payment mechanism for hospital inpatients. The DRG classification system places diseases into groups because related diseases and treatments tend to consume similar amounts of healthcare resources and incur similar amounts of cost. DRGs are used to determine reimbursement for hospitalized patients with healthcare coverage under Medicare.

Diagnostic and Statistical Manual of Mental Disorders, Fourth Edition (DSM-IV): The diagnostic coding system for substance abuse and mental health patients. *DSM-IV* is published by the American Psychiatric Association.

Diagnostic services: All diagnostic services of any type including history, physical examination, laboratory, x-ray or radiograph, and others that are performed or ordered pertinent to the patient's reasons for the encounter.

Dichotomous data: *See* nominal data

Direct obstetric death: The death of a woman resulting from obstetric complications of the pregnancy state, labor, or puerperium; from interventions, omissions, or treatment; or from a chain of events resulting from any of the above.

Disability: A physical or mental condition that makes an insured person incapable of performing one or more occupational duties either temporarily, long-term, or totally.

Disabled: Any physical or mental condition that renders an insured person unable to do work for which he or she is qualified and educated.

Discharge: *See* Inpatient discharge

Discharge date (inpatient): The year, month, and day of discharge. An inpatient discharge occurs with the termination of the room, board, and continuous nursing services, and the formal release of an inpatient by the hospital.

Discharge days: 1. *See* Length of stay. 2. *See* Total length of stay

Discharge diagnoses/list of discharge diagnoses: The complete set or list of discharge diagnoses applicable to a single patient experience, such as inpatient hospitalization.

Discharge diagnosis: Any one of the diagnoses recorded after all data accumulated in the course of a patient's hospitalization or other circumscribed episode of medical care have been studied.

Discharge transfer: The transfer of an inpatient to another healthcare institution at the time of discharge.

Discrete data: Data that contain only finite numbers. Discrete data can have only specified values.

Disposition (outpatient): The healthcare practitioner's statement of the next step(s) in the care of the patient. At a minimum, the following classification is suggested:

1. No follow-up planned (return if needed, PRN)
2. Follow-up planned or scheduled
3. Referred elsewhere (including to hospital)
4. Expired

Disposition of patient/discharge status (inpatient): A core health data element that identifies the circumstances under which the patient left the hospital. Developed by the National Committee on Vital and Health Statistics, these circumstances include:

1. Discharged Alive:

    A. Discharged to home or self care (routine discharge)
    B. Discharged/transferred to another short term general hospital for inpatient care
    C. Discharged/transferred to skilled nursing facility (SNF)
    D. Discharged/transferred to an intermediate care facility (ICF)
    E. Discharged/transferred to another type of institution for inpatient care or referred for outpatient services to another institution
    F. Discharged/transferred to home under care of organized home health services organization
    G. Discharged/transferred to home under care of a Home IV provider
    H. Left against medical advice or discontinued care

2. Expired
3. Status not stated

DME: *See* Durable medical equipment

DOA: *See* Dead on arrival

DRG: *See* Diagnosis related group

DSM-IV: *See* Diagnostic and Statistical Manual of Mental Disorders, Fourth Edition

Durable medical equipment (DME): Equipment that can endure repeated use without being subject to disposal after one-time use.

Duration of inpatient hospitalization: *See* Length of stay

E-codes (External cause of injury code): ICD-9-CM codes for the external causes of injury, poisoning, and adverse effect that explain how the injury occurred.

EDI: *See* Electronic data interchange

Education Level: The highest level, in years, within each major (primary, secondary, college, post-baccalaureate) educational system, irrespective of any certifications achieved.

Elective admission: The formal acceptance by a healthcare organization of a patient whose condition permits adequate time to schedule the availability of a suitable accommodation.

Elective surgery: Surgery that does not have to be performed immediately to prevent death or serious disability. If surgery can be scheduled at some future date, it is, by definition, elective.

Electronic data interchange (EDI): The exchange of business transaction data between organizations using electronic communications. The data format and electronic language must be standardized for both organizations.

E/M codes: *See* Evaluation and management codes

Emergency outpatient: A patient who is admitted to the emergency, accident, or equivalent service of the hospital for diagnosis and treatment of a condition that requires immediate medical, dental, or allied services.

Emergency outpatient care service: A service provided to outpatients to sustain life or prevent critical consequences and that should be performed immediately. This service is usually hospital-based.

Emergency outpatient unit (emergency department): An outpatient care unit (usually hospital-based) that provides medical services that are urgently needed to sustain life or prevent critical consequences, and that should be performed immediately.

Emergency patient: A patient admitted to the emergency room service of a hospital for diagnosis and therapy that requires immediate healthcare services.

Emergency services: Immediate evaluation and therapy rendered in emergency clinical conditions and sustained until the patient can be referred to his or her personal practitioner for further care.

Encounter: An instance of direct (usually face-to-face) interaction, regardless of the setting, between a patient and a practitioner vested with primary responsibility for diagnosing, evaluating, or treating the patient's condition, or both, or providing social worker services. Encounters do not include ancillary services visits or telephone contacts.

Episode: One or more healthcare services received by an individual during a period of relatively continuous care by healthcare practitioners in relation to a particular clinical problem or situation.

Episode of care: One or more healthcare services received by an individual during a period of relatively continuous care by healthcare providers in relation to a particular clinical problem or situation. This definition is applicable to the patient whose care for a single illness or injury is exclusively ambulatory as well as patients who use a combination of healthcare providers in relation to a particular clinical problem or situation.

Ethnic group: That cultural group with which the patient identifies him/herself either by means of recorded family data or personal preference. A patient may belong to several such groups depending upon heritage, language, nationality, or social association.

Ethnicity: The Uniform Hospital Discharge Data Set (UHDDS) provides the following categories for ethnicity:

1. Hispanic Origin (specify)

2. Other (specify)

3. Unknown/not stated

Evaluation and management (E/M) codes: CPT codes that describe patient encounters with healthcare professionals for the purpose of evaluation and management of general health status.

Exceptionally large baby: Any neonate weighing 4,500 grams or more at birth.

Extended care facility: A facility that is licensed by applicable state or local law to offer room and board, skilled nursing by a full-time registered nurse, intermediate care, or a combination of levels on a 24-hour basis.

Extreme immaturity: Birth weight of less than 1,000 grams and/or gestation of less than 28 completed weeks.

Facilities (health): Buildings, including physical plant, equipment, and supplies, necessary in the provision of health services. Major types include hospitals, nursing homes, and ambulatory care centers

Facility identification: A unique universal identification number across data systems.

Fee-for-service: A method of payment to healthcare providers whereby a payment is made for each service provided. The cost is based on the provider's estimate of the cost for services rendered.

Fee schedule: The maximum fees a plan will pay for services, primarily listed by CPT codes.

Fetal death: A death prior to the complete expulsion or extraction from its mother (in a hospital facility) of a product of human conception (fetus and placenta), irrespective of the duration of pregnancy. In accordance with the number of weeks' gestation, fetal deaths may be classified into the following categories:

Early: Less than 20 weeks' gestation, 500 grams or less.

Intermediate: 20 completed weeks' gestation, but less than 28,501 to 1,000 grams.

Late: 28 completed weeks' gestation and more than 1,001 grams.

Fetal death rate: The proportion of intermediate and/or late fetal deaths to the total number of live births, intermediate fetal deaths, and late fetal deaths during a specified period of time.

Fiscal intermediary: An organization that serves as the claims processor for Medicare hospital services.

Frequency distribution table: A table that consists of a set of classes or categories along with the numerical counts that correspond to nominal and ordinal data.

Functional status: The measure of a patient's mental and/or physical abilities. An increasingly important health measure, the functional status has been linked to medical care utilization rates. A number of scales have been developed that include:

- self-report measures, such as the listings of limitations of Activities of Daily Living (ADL), Instrumental Activities of Daily Living (IADL), and the National Health Interview Survey age-specific summary evaluation of activity limitations

- clinical assessments, such as the International Classification of Impairments, Disabilities and Handicaps (ICIDH), and the Resident Assessment Instrument (RAI) (which is widely used in nursing homes).

In addition, there are some disabilities, such as severe mental illness or blindness, where ADLs and IADLs are not sufficient measures.

Gatekeeper: The primary care physician (PCP) who participates in a comprehensive managed care plan and is responsible for the care provided to the managed care enrollee (patient).

Gender: The biological sex of the patient as recorded at the start of care.

Graph: A pictorial representation of numerical data. A graph is the best medium for presenting data for quick visualization of relationships between various factors.

Gross autopsy rate: The ratio of all inpatient autopsies to all inpatient deaths during a specified period of time.

Gross death rate: *See* death rate

HCFA: *See* Health Care Financing Administration

HCFA 1450: *See* UB-92 Uniform Bill

HCFA 1500: A standardized claim form, developed by the Health Care Financing Administration, for providers of services to bill professional fees to health carriers or third-party payers. HCFA 1500 is not used for hospital or institutional charges.

HCFA Common Procedural Coding System (HCPCS): A coding system for services and supplies composed of CPT codes, national codes developed by the Health Care Financing Administration (HCFA), and local codes developed by the fiscal intermediary.

HCPCS: *See* HCFA Common Procedural Coding System

Health: A state of complete physical, mental, and social well-being and not merely the absence of disease of infirmity.

Health Care Financing Administration (HCFA): A division of the U.S. Department of Health and Human Services responsible for Medicare healthcare policy and administration and federal participation in the Medicaid program

Healthcare practitioner: The person responsible for the services delivered to the patient.

Healthcare practitioner identification (outpatient): The unique national identification number assigned to the healthcare practitioner of record for each encounter. There may be more than one healthcare provider identified, including:

- The healthcare practitioner professionally responsible for the services, including ambulatory procedures, delivered to the patient (healthcare practitioner of record)

- The healthcare practitioner for each clinical service received by the patient, including ambulatory procedures.

Healthcare services: Processes that directly or indirectly contribute to the health and well-being of patients, such as medical, nursing, and other health-related services.

Health Insurance Portability and Accountability Act of 1996 (HIPAA): Signed into law by President Bill Clinton on August 21, 1996, this act limits exclusions for pre-existing medical conditions, prohibits discrimination against employees and dependents based on their health status, guarantees availability of health insurance to small employers, and guarantees renewability of insurance to all employees regardless of size. *Portability* means that individuals maintain their health coverage even though they switch employers or health plans.

Health maintenance organization (HMO): An organization that provides health coverage to voluntary enrollees in return for prepayment of a set fee, regardless of the services used. An HMO has management responsibility for providing comprehensive healthcare services on a prepayment basis to voluntarily enrolled persons within a designated population.

HMOs focus on preventive medicine and managing premiums or capitated rates by payers for each person enrolled, which is based on a projection of what the typical patient will cost. If enrollees cost more than the projection, the HMO could suffer losses. If the enrollees cost less, the HMO profits. This gives the HMO incentive to control costs. Payers include employers, insurance companies, government agencies, and other groups representing covered lives.

Under the Federal HMO Act, an entity must have three characteristics to call itself an HMO:

1. An organized system for providing healthcare or otherwise assuring healthcare delivery in a geographic area;

2. An agreed upon set of basic and supplemental health maintenance and treatment services; and

3. A voluntarily enrolled group of people. HMOs must also meet many rules and regulations required at the state level.

There are four types of HMO's:

1. *Staff Model HMO:* The physicians are hired, paid, and considered employees of the HMO.

2. *Individual Practice Association (IPA):* The physicians are paid on a fee-for-services basis by the HMO. The HMO contracts with an organized group of physicians who come together for contracting purposes but retain their individual practices. They are not considered employees of the HMO; however, the HMO pays the physicians from a fund for this purpose. The IPA physicians provide care to HMO members from their private offices and continue to see their fee-for-service patients.

3. *Group Model HMO:* The HMO contracts with a multi-specialty physician group to provide services to HMO members. The providers usually agree to devote a fixed percentage of time to the HMO.

4. *Network Model HMO:* Similar to a Group HMO, but the HMO contracts for services with two or more medical groups.

Health Plan Employer Data and Information Set (HEDIS): The result of a coordinated development effort by the National Committee for Quality Assurance to provide performance measures that gives employers some objective information with which to evaluate health plans and hold them accountable. HEDIS helps ensure that plans and purchasers of care are speaking the same language when they are comparing value and accountability.

HEDIS: *See* Health Plan Employer Data and Information Set

HIPAA: *See* Health Insurance Portability and Accountability Act of 1996

Histogram: The graph form used for the display of frequency distributions for continuous numerical data (interval or ratio data).

HMO: *See* Health maintenance organization

HMO Act: A 1973 federal act outlining requirements for federal qualification of health maintenance organizations, consisting of legal and organizational structures, financial strength requirements, marketing provisions, and healthcare delivery. HMOs seek the voluntary status of "federally qualified" in order to gain credibility with employers, as well as the chance to gain covered lives from dual-choice mandates that require employee access to such plans.

HMO referral: *See* Source of admission

Home care program: A program through which a blend of health and social services is provided to individuals and families in their places of residence for the purpose of promoting, maintaining, or restoring health or of minimizing the effects of illness an disability.

Home healthcare: Clinical care provided or supervised by a practitioner, administered at the patient's home or place of residence, thus allowing the patient to remain at home during an illness. Home healthcare also addresses care for people with permanent alterations in their health or functional status.

Hospice: A program emphasizing psychosocial support and home physical care, with inpatient care when needed, for terminally ill patients and their families.

Hospital: An establishment with an organized medical staff with permanent facilities that include inpatient beds and continuous medical/nursing services and that provide diagnosis and treatment for patients.

Hospital ambulatory care: All hospital-directed preventive, therapeutic, and rehabilitative services provided by physicians and their surrogates to patients who are not hospital inpatients.

This definition refers only to those services for which the hospital is responsible, whether rendered at the hospital facility (hospital-based) or at another facility where the care is coordinated by the hospital, such as a neighborhood health center. The services of physicians who rent space in a hospital for their offices, or groups such as visiting nurses associations who use the hospital for their headquarters, are not considered part of hospital ambulatory care.

Hospital autopsy: The postmortem examination, wherever performed (by a hospital pathologist or by a physician to whom the responsibility has been delegated), of the body of a person who has at some time been a hospital patient.

Hospital autopsy rate (adjusted): The proportion of death of hospital patients following which the bodies of the deceased persons are available for autopsy and hospital autopsies performed. See also Available for hospital autopsy.

Hospital-based ambulatory care center: An organized hospital facility providing non-emergency medical or dental services to patients who are not assigned to a bed as inpatients during the time services are rendered. An emergency department in which services are provided to non-emergency patients does not constitute an organized ambulatory care center.

Hospital-based outpatient care: A subset of ambulatory care that utilizes the hospital staff, equipment, and resources to render preventive or corrective healthcare, or both.

Hospital fetal death: Death prior to the complete expulsion or extraction from its mother, in a hospital facility, of a product of human conception (fetus and placenta), irrespective of the duration of pregnancy. The death is indicated by the fact that after such expulsion or extraction, the fetus does not breathe or show any other evidence of life such as beating of the heart, pulsation of the umbilical cord, or definite movement of voluntary muscles. Fetal deaths are divided into the following categories:

Early Fetal Death: Less than 20 weeks' gestation, 500 grams or less

Intermediate Fetal Death: 20 completed weeks' gestation but less than 28,501 to 1,000 grams

Late Fetal Death: 28 completed weeks' gestation and more than 1,001 grams

Hospital identification: A unique institutional number within a data collection system.

Hospital inpatient: A hospital patient who is provided with room, board, and continuous general nursing service in an area of the hospital where patients generally stay at least overnight.

Hospital inpatient autopsy: The postmortem examination performed in a hospital facility (by a hospital pathologist or by a physician to whom the responsibility has been delegated) of the body of a patient who died during inpatient hospitalization.

Hospital inpatient beds: Accommodations with supporting services (such as food, laundry, and housekeeping) for hospital inpatients, excluding those for the newborn nursery. Incubators and bassinets in nurseries for premature or sick newborn infants are considered inpatient beds.

Hospitalization: *See* Inpatient hospitalization

Hospital live birth: The complete expulsion or extraction from the mother, in a hospital facility, of a product of human conception, irrespective of the duration of pregnancy, which, after such expulsion or extraction, breathes or shows any other evidence of life, such as beating of the heart, pulsation of the umbilical cord, or definite movement of voluntary muscles whether or not the umbilical cord has been cut or the placenta is attached.

Hospital newborn bassinets: Accommodations with supporting services (such as food, laundry, and housekeeping) for hospital newborn inpatients. These include bassinets, incubators, and isolettes in the newborn nursery.

Hospital newborn inpatient: A hospital patient born in the hospital at the beginning of the current hospitalization. This definition acknowledges the fact that infants born in a hospital, occupying beds (usually bassinets), and receiving medical services are hospital inpatients. However, they are atypical inpatients and their hospital experiences and the arrangements for their care are so different from those of other patients that they are usually considered separately. Infants who are born at home or on the way to the hospital are classified as hospital inpatients, not as hospital newborn inpatients.

Hospital outpatient: A hospital patient who receives services in one or more of the facilities of the hospital when he or she is not currently an inpatient or a home care patient.

Hospital outpatient care unit: An organized unit of a hospital, with facilities and medical services exclusively or primarily for patients who are generally ambulatory and who do not currently require or are not currently receiving services as an inpatient of the hospital.

Hospital patient: A person receiving healthcare services for which the hospital has a responsibility for the healthcare.

ICD-9-CM: *See* International Classification of Disease, Ninth Edition, Clinical Modification

ICF: *See* Intermediate care facility

IDS: *See* Integrated delivery system

Indirect obstetric death: The death of a woman resulting from a previously existing disease (or a disease that developed during pregnancy, labor, or the puerperium) that was not due to obstetric causes, although the physiologic effects of pregnancy were partially responsible for the death.

Individual provider: A health professional who delivers (or is professionally responsible for) services delivered to a patient, who is exercising independent judgment in the care of the patient, and who is not under the immediate supervision of another healthcare professional.

Induced termination of pregnancy: The purposeful interruption of an intrauterine pregnancy with the intention other than to produce a live-born infant, and which does not result in a live birth. This definition excludes management of prolonged retention of products of conception following fetal death.

Infant death: The death of a liveborn infant at any time from the moment of birth to the end of the first year of life (364 days, 23 hours, 59 minutes from the moment of birth).

Infant mortality rate: The ratio of all infant deaths (neonatal and postneonatal) to the total number of live births during a specified period of time.

Inpatient: A hospital patient receiving healthcare services and who is provided room, board, and continuous nursing services in a unit or area of the hospital.

Inpatient admission: The formal acceptance by a hospital of a patient who is to be provided with room, board, and continuous nursing service in an area of the hospital where patients generally stay at least overnight.

Inpatient days of stay: *See* Length of stay.

Inpatient discharge: The termination of a period of inpatient hospitalization through the formal release of the inpatient by the hospital.

Inpatient hospitalization: A period in a person's life during which he or she is an inpatient in a single hospital without interruption, except by possible intervening leaves of absence.

Inpatient service day: A unit of measure denoting the services received by one inpatient in one 24-hour period.

Insurance: A purchased contract (policy) in which the purchaser (insured) is protected from loss by the insurer's agreeing to reimburse for such loss.

Integrated delivery system (IDS): An integrated financing and delivery system that uses a panel of providers, selected on the basis of quality and cost management criteria, to furnish members with comprehensive health services. An IDS is also known as an *integrated medical system* or *integrated health system.*

Intensity of service/severity of illness criteria: The standard criteria used by a medical review entity to justify admission to an inpatient facility.

Intermediate care facility: An institution that provides health-related care and services to individuals who do not require the degree of care or treatment that a hospital or skilled nursing facility is designated to provide, but who, because of their physical or mental condition, require care and services.

International Classification of Disease, Ninth Edition, Clinical Modification (ICD-9-CM): A statistical grouping of similar diagnoses and procedures used for coding purposes. The ninth and current edition has been adapted for use in the United States. Its conventions include special terms, punctuation marks, abbreviations, or symbols used as shorthand in the ICD coding system to efficiently communicate special instructions to the coder. If the conventions are ignored, the code number established may be incorrect.

Interval data: Data that includes units of equal size, such as intelligence quotient (IQ) results.

Intrahospital transfer: A change in medical care unit, medical staff unit, or responsible physician during hospitalization.

JCAHO: *See* Joint Commission on Accreditation of Health Care Organizations

Joint Commission on Accreditation of Health Care Organizations (JCAHO): A private, not-for-profit organization that evaluates and accredits hospitals and other healthcare organizations providing home care, mental healthcare, ambulatory care, and long-term care services. JCAHO was established in 1951 to enhance the quality of care provided by hospitals and other organizations by monitoring and implementing standards of practice that organizations must achieve to receive recognition and accreditation. The Joint Commission revises its standards every year, but reviews organizations approximately every three years. These reviews involve JCAHO medical and administrative representatives who analyze the organization's policies, patient records, credentialing procedures, and quality assurance programs.

Leave of absence: The authorized absence of an inpatient from a hospital or other facility for a specified period of time occurring after admission and prior to discharge.

Length of stay (LOS): The total number of patient days for an inpatient episode, calculated by subtracting the date of admission from the date of discharge. If a patient is admitted and discharged on the same date, the LOS is one day.

Level of service: The relative intensity of services given when a physician provides one-on-one services for a patient (such as minimal, brief, limited, or intermediate). The term can also refer to the various levels of service provided by a healthcare organization (for example: ambulatory surgery, tertiary).

Licensed practitioners: An individual at any level of professional specialization who requires a public license/certification to practice the delivery of care to patients. A practitioner can also be a provider.

Line graph: A graph used to illustrate the relationship between continuous quantities.

Living arrangement: A data element that denotes whether the patient lives alone or with whom. The categories for living arrangement are defined by ASTM as:

- Alone
- With spouse
- With significant other/life partner
- With children
- With parent or guardian
- With relatives
- With nonrelatives
- Unknown/not stated

Location or address of encounter (outpatient): The full address and zip code (nine digits preferred) for the location at which care was received from the healthcare practitioner of record. The address should be in sufficient detail to allow for the calculation of state, county, and metropolitan statistics.

Longitudinal patient record: A permanent, coordinated patient record of significant information listed in chronological sequence. This record may include all historical data collected or be retrieved as a user-designated synopsis of significant demographic, genetic, clinical, and environmental facts and events maintained within an automated system.

Long-term care: Healthcare rendered in a non-acute care facility and to a patient in resident status or non-resident status. Such illness is not severe enough to require an acute care facility, but is in need of continual supervision and assistance by healthcare practitioners.

Long-term care facility: An organization that provides nursing care and related services for residents who require medical, nursing, rehabilitation, or subacute care services. Such a facility may be certified for participation in the Medicare or Medicaid program as a skilled nursing facility or other nursing facility.

LOS: *See* length of stay

Low birth weight neonate: Any neonate, regardless of gestational age, whose weight at birth is less than 2,500 grams.

Major diagnostic category (MDC): The initial broad classification of diagnoses to which a patient is assigned when determining a DRG. MDCs are typically grouped by body system.

Managed care: A generic term for a payment system that manages cost, quality, and access to healthcare. Managed care systems control costs by presetting reimbursement amounts and regulating patient access to participating physicians and healthcare institutions.

Marital status: The marital state of the patient at the start of care. Marital status categories include:

- *Married:* A person currently married. Common law marriage is classified as married.

    A. Living together
    B. Not living together

- *Never Married:* A person who has never been married or whose only marriages have been annulled

- *Widowed:* A person whose spouse has died and not remarried

- *Divorced:* A person legally divorced and not remarried

- *Separated:* Married persons living apart except institutionalized.

- *Unknown/not stated*

Maternal death: The death of any woman, from any cause, related to or aggravated by pregnancy or its management (regardless of duration or site of pregnancy), but not from accidental or incidental causes.

MDC: *See* Major diagnostic category

MDS: *See* Minimum data set

Mean: An arithmetic average.

Measures of central tendency: A typical or average number that is descriptive of the entire collection of data or specific population.

Median: The midpoint (center) of the distribution of values.

Medicaid: A jointly funded program between state and federal governments to provide healthcare to low-income people. Originally titled the medical assistance program, Medicaid was established in 1966 by Title XIX, an amendment of the Social Security Act of 1935.

Medical care unit: An assemblage of inpatient beds (or newborn bassinets), related facilities, and assigned personnel that provide service to a defined and limited class of patients according to their particular medical care needs.

Medical classification system: A method of arranging related disease entities into groups for the reporting of quantitative data for statistical purposes.

Medical consultation: *See* Consultation

Medical nomenclature: A recognized system of preferred terminology for naming disease processes.

Medical staff organization (MSO): A self-governing entity that operates as a responsible extension of the governing body and exists for the purpose of providing patient care.

Medical staff unit: One of the departments, divisions, or specialties into which the organized medical staff of a hospital is divided in order to fulfill medical staff responsibility.

Medicare: A federally funded program that provides payment for healthcare services for the elderly and certain categories of illnesses. Medicare was established in 1966 by Title VXIII, an amendment to the Social Security Act of 1935.

Medicare Conditions of Participation (COPs): Requirements that institutional providers (such as hospitals, skilled nursing facilities, and home health agencies) must meet to be allowed to receive payments for Medicare patients.

Medicare discharge: Medicare patients are considered discharged when they:

- are formally released from the hospital;
- die in the hospital; or
- are transferred to another hospital or unit excluded from the prospective payment system.

Medications prescribed: A description of all medications prescribed or provided by the healthcare practitioner at the encounter (for outpatients) or given on discharge to the patient (for inpatients). This description includes (where possible) the national drug code, dosage, strength, and total amount prescribed.

Minimum data set (MDS): A common core of data elements collected for long-term care residents. This information, which has been collected in nursing homes for years, is the cornerstone on which all long-term care patient documentation and reimbursement rests. Beginning in June 1998, the federal government has required electronic collection and transmission of MDS data.

Mode: The most recurring or most frequent value in a given set of data.

Morbidity: 1. The state of being diseased (including illness, injury, or deviations from normal health). 2. The number of sick persons or cases of disease in relationship to a specific population.

Mortality: The death rate in relationship to a specific population.

Most significant diagnosis: The diagnosis that describes the most important or significant condition of a patient regarding his or her health, medical care, and use of the hospital. This diagnosis is often, but not necessarily, the principal diagnosis.

MSO: *See* Medical staff organization

Multiple birth: *See* Source of admission

National Committee for Quality Assurance (NCQA): An accreditation organization that evaluates and reports on the quality of managed care plans. This information enables purchasers and consumers of managed healthcare to distinguish among plans on the basis of quality. To assist in performance measurement, the NCQA developed the Health Employer Data Information Set (HEDIS), a set of standardized measures.

NCQA: *See* National Committee for Quality Assurance

Neonatal death: The death of a liveborn infant within the first 27 days, 23 hours, and 59 minutes from the moment of birth.

Neonatal period: The period of an infant's life from the hour of birth through the first 27 days, 23 hours, and 59 minutes of life. During this period, the infant is referred to as a newborn infant. The neonatal period is divided into three subcategories:

Neonatal Period I: From the hour of birth through 23 hours and 59 minutes

Neonatal Period II: From the beginning of the 24th hour of life through 6 days, 23 hours, and 59 minutes

Neonatal Period III: From the beginning of the 7th day through 27 days, 23 hours, and 59 minutes

Net autopsy rate: The ratio of all inpatient autopsies to all inpatient deaths minus unautopsied coroners' or medical examiner's cases during a specified period of time.

Net death rate: The death rate excluding deaths under 48 hours of admission.

Newborn bassinet count: The number of available hospital newborn bassinets, both occupied and vacant, on any given day.

Nomenclature: A system of names used in any science or art.

Nominal data: One of the simplest types of data where the values fall into unordered categories. Also called dichotomous data.

Non-licensed practitioner: An individual without a public license/certification who is supervised by a licensed/certified individual in delivering care to patients.

Normal distribution: A distribution that would display a normal pattern, with most of the measurements near the center of the frequency.

Nosocomial infection: An infection that is acquired by an individual while receiving care or services in a healthcare organization.

Nosocomial infection rate: The ratio describing the number of patients with nosocomial infections divided by the number of patients at risk of developing nosocomial infections. Rates may be stratified by taking into account certain factors that may predispose a specified group of patients to an increased risk of acquiring a nosocomial infection.

Not-for-profit: An organizational category that implies that the organization will use its excess funds after expenses to enhance services to the community the organization serves rather than distribute the excess to owners of the organization.

Numerical data: Data that include discrete data and continuous data.

Nursing facility: A comprehensive term for a long-term care facility that provides nursing care and related services for residents who require medical, nursing, or rehabilitative care. A sufficient number of nursing personnel must be employed on a 24-hour basis to provide care to residents according to the care plan.

OASIS: *See* Outcomes and Assessment Information Set

Observation patient: A patient who presents with a medical condition with a significant degree of instability and patient disability and who needs to be monitored, evaluated, and assessed whether they should be admitted to inpatient status or discharged for care in another setting.

Medicare guidelines note that this type of patient should be evaluated against standard inpatient criteria. If the patient is expected to need hospital care for more than 24 hours, they should be admitted as an inpatient. If not, then plans should be made for discharge to an appropriate setting. Inpatient status is not determined by the length of stay but by the physician's intent at the time of admission.

An observation patient can occupy special beds set aside for this purpose or may occupy beds in any unit in a hospital (for example, emergency, medical unit, or obstetrics). The length of the observation period should not be longer than approximately 36 to 48 hours. Patients in the observation status are usually billed on an hourly basis.

Occasion of service: A specified identifiable instance of an act of service involved in the care of a patient or consumer that is not an encounter. Occasions of service may be the result of an encounter (for example, tests or procedures ordered as part of an encounter).

Occupancy percent/ratio: *See* Bed occupancy ratio

Occupation: The employment, business, or a course of action in which the patient is engaged.

Occupational health: The degree to which an employee is able to function at an optimum level of well-being at work as reflected by productivity, work attendance, disability compensation claims, and employment longevity.

Occupational health services: Health services involving the physical, mental, and social well-being of individuals in relation to their work and working environment.

OCE: *See* Outpatient Code Editor

Operating clinician identification: The unique national identification number assigned to the clinician who performed the principal procedure.

Operating physician/clinician: The clinician who performed the principal procedure.

Operating room: An area of a hospital equipped and staffed to provide facilities and personnel services for the performance of surgical procedures.

Operation: *See* Surgical operation

Ordinal data: A type of data where the values are in ordered categories or are ranked.

Organized medical staff: A formal organization of physicians (or other professionals, such as dentists) with the delegated authority and responsibility to maintain proper standards of medical care and to plan for continued betterment of that care.

Osteopath: A physician licensed to practice in osteopathy. The philosophy of osteopathy focuses on the whole body, with emphasis on prevention, health, and the interrelationship of structure and function.

Other diagnoses (inpatient): All conditions that coexist at the time of admission, or develop subsequently, which affect the treatment received and/or the length of stay. Diagnoses that refer to an earlier episode that have no bearing on the current hospital or nursing home stay are to be excluded. Diagnoses to be coded include conditions that affect patient care by requiring clinical evaluation, therapeutic treatment, diagnostic procedures, extended length of hospital or nursing home stay, or increased care and/or monitoring.

Other diagnoses (outpatient): All conditions that coexist at the time of admission, develop subsequently, or affect the treatment received and/or length of stay. These conditions should be recorded to the highest documented level of specificity.

Outcome: The end result of healthcare treatment; the performance (or nonperformance) of one or more processes, services, or activities carried out by healthcare providers. A *patient health outcome* represents the cumulative effect of one or more processes at a defined time (for example, survival to discharge following a gunshot wound to the chest or an acute myocardial infarction).

Outcomes and Assessment Information Set (OASIS): A standard core assessment data tool developed to measure the outcomes of adult patients receiving home health services. OASIS provides data that help identify appropriate clinical outcomes and reimbursement rates and pave the way for a home health prospective payment system.

Outcomes assessment: An evaluation that measures the actual outcomes of patient care and service against predetermined criteria (expected outcomes). This evaluation is based on the premise that care is delivered in order to bring about certain results.

Outcomes management: A proactive approach to improving healthcare outcomes by using information gained through monitoring activities to improve clinical decision making and care delivery.

Outcomes measurement: The process of systematically tracking a patient's clinical treatment and responses to that treatment, including measures of morbidity and functional status, for the purpose of improving care.

Outcomes monitoring: The ongoing measurement of outcomes indicators over time to support hypotheses regarding the causes of the outcomes.

Outliers: Extreme statistical values. In healthcare reimbursement, the term refers to patients statistically outside the norm, such as those who require an unusually long hospital stay (*stay outliers*) or who generate unusually high costs (*cost outliers*).

Out-of-pocket: Moneys that the patient pays directly to a healthcare provider.

Outpatient: A patient who receives care without being admitted for inpatient or resident care.

Outpatient code editor (OCE): A software program, developed by the Health Care Financing Administration, that analyzes outpatient claims to detect incorrect billing and coding data and to determine whether ambulatory surgery center payment limitations apply. Medicare carriers use the OCE to test the validity of ICD-9-CM coding and conduct compatibility edits.

Outpatient unit: An outpatient care unit that is organized into sections (clinics). The number of sections depends on the size and degree of departmentalization of the medical or clinic staff, available facilities, type of service needed in the community, and the needs of the patients for whom it accepts responsibility.

Outpatient visit: The visit of an outpatient to one or more units or facilities located in, or directed by the provider maintaining, the outpatient healthcare services (such as a clinic, physician's office, or hospital/medical center).

Palliative care: Healthcare services that relieve or alleviate patient symptoms or discomforts, such as pain or nausea. Palliative care is not curative.

Partial hospital program: Facilities of the hospital are regularly used on a scheduled care basis for a substantial number of daytime or nighttime hours.

Partial hospitalization: A hospital term for patients who spend limited time in the hospital setting, typically as part of a transition program to a less intense level of service. Psychiatric, drug, and alcohol facilities frequently use partial hospitalization to help a patient reenter the community, return to work, and assume family responsibilities. The patient may spend one or more days a week or one or more nights at the facility.

Patient: A person who is receiving or has received healthcare services, including a deceased person.

PCP: *See* Primary care physician

Patient health outcome: *See* Outcome

Patient health record: The primary legal record documenting the healthcare services provided to a person, in any aspect of healthcare delivery. The term includes routine clinical or office records, records of care in any health-related setting, preventive care, lifestyle evaluation, research protocols, special study records and various clinical databases.

As the repository of information about a single patient, the health record is generated by healthcare professionals as a direct result of interaction with a patient or with individuals who have personal knowledge of the patient (or with both). The record contains information about the patient and other individuals as they relate to the health of the patient (for example, family history or caregiver support).

Patient record system: The set of components that form the mechanism by which patient records are created, used, stored, and retrieved. A patient record system is usually located within a healthcare provider/practitioner setting. The system includes people, data, rules and procedures, processing and storage devices (such as paper and pen, hardware, and software), and communications and support functions.

Patient's expected sources of payment: Regardless of payment method, the *primary source* is expected to be responsible for the largest percentage of the patient's current bill. The *secondary source,* if any, is responsible for the next largest percentage of the bill. Methods of payment include:

- Self-pay
- Worker's Compensation
- Medicare
- Medicaid
- Maternal and Child Health
- Other government payments
- Blue Cross
- Insurance Companies
- No charge (free, charity, special research, or teaching)
- Other
- Unknown/not stated

Pediatric patient: A patient usually under the age of 14.

Pediatric service: A service providing diagnosis and treatment of patients usually under the age of 14.

Peer review: An evaluation of professional performance by other people of equal standing within the same profession.

Peer review organization (PRO): A medical review entity under contract to the Health Care Financing Administration to monitor the medical necessity, quality, and appropriateness of services provided to Medicare beneficiaries.

Per case: A method of billing in which services are charged based on the total service being rendered rather than by each component of the service. For example, charging for "transplantation services" when all of the following have been performed: the organ has been procured, the transplant has been made, and aftercare has been rendered.

Percentage: A value computed on the basis of the whole divided into 100 parts.

Percentage of occupancy/percent occupancy: *See* Bed occupancy ratio

Per diem: An established payment for a day's worth of services.

Per diem rate: The cost per day, derived by dividing total costs by the number of inpatient days of care given. Per diem costs are an average and do not reflect the true cost for each patient. Under DRG's, the per diem rate is the payment made for each day of stay to the hospital at which a DRG patient is transferred. The rate is determined by dividing the full DRG payment by the geometric mean length of stay (GMLOS) for the DRG. The payment rate for the first day of stay is twice the per diem rate; subsequent days are paid at the per diem rate.

Perinatal death: An all-inclusive term referring to both stillborn infants and neonatal deaths.

Personal/unique identifier: The unique name or numeric identifier that will set apart information for an individual person for research and administrative purposes.

Point-of-care documentation: Data entry at the time and location of service.

Point-of-care system: A system of data capture at the site where the service of care is provided.

Point of service: A component of managed care plans in which the patient is required to use a primary care physician (gatekeeper) who is responsible for the care provided.

Postneonatal death: The death of a live-born infant from 28 days to the end of the first year of life (364 days, 23 hours, 59 minutes from the moment of birth).

Postneonatal mortality rate: The number of deaths that occur from 28 days to 364 days after birth per 1,000 live births.

Postoperative death rate: The ratio of deaths within ten days after surgery to the total number of operations performed during a specified period of time.

Postoperative infection rate: The ratio of all infections in clean surgical cases to the number of surgical operations.

Post-term infant: A fetus or infant with a gestation period of 294 days or more (42 completed weeks or more).

Post-term neonate: Any neonate whose birth occurs from the beginning of the first day (295th day) of the 43rd week following onset of the last menstrual period.

PPO: *See* Preferred provider organization

PPS: *See* Prospective payment system

Pre-existing condition: Any disease, injury, or condition identified as having occurred before a specific date.

Preferred provider organization (PPO): A contractual agreement between healthcare providers (professional and/or institutional) and employers, insurance carriers, or third party administrators to provide healthcare services to a defined population at established fees which may or may not be a discount from usual and customary or reasonable charges.

Pregnancy termination: The birth of a live born or stillborn infant or the expulsion or extraction of a dead fetus or other products of conception from the mother.

Premature delivery: *See* Source of Admission

Preterm infant: An infant with a birth weight between 1,000-2,499 grams and/or a gestation between 28-37 completed weeks.

Preterm neonate: Any neonate whose birth occurs through the end of the last day of the 38th week (266th day) following onset of the last menstrual period.

Primary care: The care provided at first contact with the healthcare provider in an ambulatory care setting. Primary care is continuous and comprehensive.

Primary care physician (PCP): The physician who makes an initial diagnosis and referral and retains control over the patient and utilization of services both in and outside the plan.

Primary diagnosis: *See* Principal diagnosis

Primary patient record/primary record of care: *See* Patient health record

Principal diagnosis (inpatient): A statement of the condition established after study to be chiefly responsible for occasioning the admission of the patient to the hospital or nursing home for care.

Principal procedure (inpatient): The single diagnosis that was performed for definitive treatment, rather than one performed for diagnostic or exploratory purposes or was necessary to take care of a complication. If there appear to be two procedures that are principal, then the one most related to the principal diagnosis should be selected as the principal procedure.

PRO: *See* Peer review organization

Procedural risk: This term refers to a professionally recognized risk that a given procedure may induce some functional impairment, injury, morbidity, or even death.

Procedures and services (outpatient): All procedures and services of any type (including history, physical examination, laboratory, x-ray or radiograph, and others) that are performed pertinent to the patient's reasons for the encounter; all therapeutic services performed at the time of the encounter; and all preventive services and procedures performed at the time of the encounter.

Proportion: A type of ratio in which the elements included in the numerator must also be included in the denominator.

Prospective payment system (PPS): The system set forth in the *1983 Amendments to the Social Security Act* (PL.98-21) for Medicare payments for hospital inpatient services based on diagnosis related groups (DRGs). *See also* Diagnosis related groups

Provider: A general term for all providers of healthcare. ASTM defines a provider as: A business entity that furnished healthcare to a consumer; it includes a professionally licensed practitioner who is authorized to operate a healthcare delivery facility.

Psychiatric hospital: A hospital that provides diagnostic and treatment services to patients with mental or emotional disorders.

Race: The major biological class to which the patient belongs as a result of a pedigree analysis or with which the patient identifies him/herself in cases where the data are not conclusive. The categories for race include:

- American Indian/Eskimo/Aleut
- Asian or Pacific Islander (specify)
- Black
- White
- Other (specify)
- Unknown/not stated

RAI: *See* Resident assessment instrument

Range: The difference between the largest and smallest values in a frequency distribution.

Ranked data: A type of ordinal data where the group of observations are first arranged from highest to lowest according to magnitude and then assigned numbers that correspond to each observation's place in the sequence.

Rate: A ratio in which there is a distinct relationship between the numerator and denominator. A measure of time is often an intrinsic part of the denominator. The denominator often implies a large base population.

Ratio: A calculation found by dividing one quantity by another. A ratio is a general term that can include a number of specific measures, such as proportion, percentage, and rate.

Ratio data: Data that may be displayed by units of equal size that can be placed on a scale starting with zero, and thus be able to be manipulated mathematically (for example, 0, 5, 10, 15, 20).

Referenced diagnostic services: Hospitals may provide laboratory resources to physicians in the community. Specimens, such as blood or tissue, may be sent to the laboratory for examination. The hospital does not have a relationship with the patient but it does provide a service to the community. A count of the lab activity is maintained, but the individuals whose specimens are analyzed are not considered outpatients if the only activity is to receive a specimen and test it.

Referred outpatient: An outpatient who is provided special diagnostic or therapeutic service of the hospital for diagnosis or treatment on an ambulatory basis. The responsibility for medical care remains with the referring physician.

Rehabilitation: The processes of treatment and education that lead a disabled person to achievement of maximum independence and function and a personal sense of well-being.

Residence: The full address and zip code (nine digit zip code, if available) of a patient's usual residence.

Residency program: An accredited program whereby a hospital sponsors graduate medical education for physicians in training. Residencies in the clinical divisions of medicine, surgery, and other special fields provide advanced training in preparation for the practice of a specialty.

Resident: A term commonly used as a synonym for *patient,* especially in long-term care.

Resident assessment instrument (RAI): An assessment instrument used by long-term care facilities for HCFA's minimum data set. *See also* Minimum data set

Resident care facility: A residential facility that provides regular and emergency health services, when needed, and appropriate supporting services on a regular basis.

Residential arrangement: The place where an individual resides on a regular basis. The categories for residential arrangement include:

- Own home or apartment
- Residence where health, disability, or aging related services or supervision are available
- Other residential setting where no services are provided
- Nursing home or other health facility
- Other institutional setting (such as a prison)
- Homeless or homeless shelter
- Unknown/not stated

Residential care: Care (including lodging and board) provided in a protective environment to patients (including mentally retarded, chemically dependent, elderly, mentally ill, or those who need assisted living) who are not in an acute phase of illness and would be capable of self-preservation during a disaster. There is minimum supervision and little or no formal program activity. This type of care does not include medical, nursing, or rehabilitative services.

Residential care facility: A live-in facility that provides custodial care to persons who are not able to live independently because of their physical, mental, or emotional condition.

Resource-based relative value scale (RVRVS): A classification system that assigns a weight to procedures and services (CPT codes) together based on resources used to determine physician reimbursement rates.

Resource utilization group (RUG): Using resident information collected in the minimum data set, patients are classified into one of 44 possible RUG categories, each with a corresponding per diem reimbursement rate. *See also* Minimum data set

Respite care: Short-term care to individuals in the home or institution that provides temporary relief to the family home caregiver. This care may be provided during the day or overnight.

Revenue: The charges generated from providing healthcare services.

Revenue code: A three-digit number representing a specific accommodation, ancillary service, or billing calculation required for Medicare billing.

Risk management: Activities intended to minimize the potential for injuries to occur in a facility and to anticipate and respond to ensuing liabilities for injuries that occur.

RUG: *See* Resource utilization group

RVRVS: *See* Resource-based relative value scale

Satellite clinic: A primary care facility, owned and operated by a hospital or other organization, that is located in an area convenient to the patients or in an area closer to a specific patient population.

School special education: Specifically designed instruction provided by qualified teachers within the context of school, aimed at the acquisition of academic, vocational, language, social, and self-care skills. This instruction includes adapted physical education and the use of specialized techniques to overcome intrinsic learning deficits.

Secondary care: A general term for healthcare services provided by a specialist at the request of the primary care physician.

Secondary diagnosis: A statement of those conditions coexisting during a hospital episode that affect the treatment received or the length of stay.

Secondary patient record: A record, derived from the primary record, that contains selected data elements to aid nonclinical persons (that is, those not involved in direct patient care) in patient care support, evaluation, or advancement. *Patient care support* refers to administration, regulation, and payment functions. *Patient care evaluation* refers to quality assurance, utilization review, and medical or legal audits. *Patient care advancement* refers to research. These records are often combined to form a *secondary database* (for example, an insurance claims database.)

Self-pay: A payer category in which the patient or patient's family will pay the bill for care, rather than a third-party payer (such as an insurance company).

Self-reported health status: A method of measuring health status in which a person rates his or her own general health (for example, using a five-category classification: excellent, very good, good, fair, or poor). Used in the National Health Interview Survey and many other studies, this method and has been shown to be predictive of morbidity, mortality, and future healthcare use. The self-evaluation is typically collected in an interview setting at first clinical visit and periodically updated, at least annually. Although the documentation of health status has been shown to precipitate the demand for healthcare and help determine the prognosis, there is currently no consensus on how its definition should be standardized. Additional evaluation and testing are needed on standardizing the health status element. At the present time, standards-setting organizations should assign place holder(s) for this element.

Services: Services are acts performed by certain persons on behalf of other persons. In addition to services, healthcare involves the linking of personal relationships (such as patient-physician) and organized arrangements (such as health maintenance organizations) through which personal health services are made available and delivered. Healthcare also includes attention to the supply and availability of persons qualified to perform services and the facilities they need to implement these services.

Services classification: Functionally autonomous units (departments, services, or divisions) of the medical staff organization in an individual hospital.

Severity of illness system: A database, established from coded data on diseases and operations, used in the hospital for planning and research purposes.

Sheltered employment: Employment provided in a special industry or workshop for the physically, mentally, emotionally, or developmentally handicapped.

Short-stay patient: A patient admitted to the hospital for an intended stay of less than 24 hours. A short-stay patient is considered to be an outpatient and not included in inpatient hospital census statistics.

Significant procedure: A procedure that is surgical in nature or carries a procedural risk or carries an anesthetic risk or requires specialized training. Surgery includes incision, excision, amputation, introduction, endoscopy, repair, destruction, suture, and manipulation.

Skilled nursing facility: An institution with an organized professional staff and permanent facilities, including inpatient beds, that provides continuous nursing and other health-related, psychosocial, and personal services to patients who are not in an acute phase of illness but who primarily require continued care on an inpatient basis.

Sliding scale fee: A method of billing in which the cost of healthcare services are based on the patient's ability to pay.

Solo practice: A practice in which the physician is self-employed and is legally the sole owner.

Source of admission: The point from which a patient enters a healthcare organization. The categories of source of admission include:

- Physician referral

    Inpatient: The patient was admitted to the facility upon the recommendation of his or her personal physician.

    Outpatient: The patient was referred to the facility for outpatient or referenced diagnostic services by his or her personal physician, or the patient independently requested outpatient services (self-referral).

- Clinic referral

    Inpatient: The patient was admitted to the facility upon recommendation of the facility's clinic physician.

Outpatient: The patient was referred to the facility for outpatient or referenced diagnostic services by the facility's clinic or other outpatient department physician.

- HMO referral

Inpatient: The patient was admitted to the facility upon the recommendation of a health maintenance organization physician.

Outpatient: The patient was referred to the facility for outpatient or referenced diagnostic services by a health maintenance physician.

- Transfer from a hospital

Inpatient: The patient was admitted to the hospital facility as a transfer from an acute care facility where he or she was an inpatient.

Outpatient: The patient was referred to the facility for outpatient or referenced diagnostic services by a physician of another acute care facility.

- Transfer from a skilled nursing facility

Inpatient: The patient was admitted to the facility as a transfer from a skilled nursing facility where he or she was an inpatient.

Outpatient: The patient was referred to the facility for outpatient or referenced diagnostic services by a physician of the skilled nursing facility where he or she is an inpatient.

- Transfer from another healthcare facility

Inpatient: The patient was admitted to the facility as a transfer from another healthcare facility other than an acute care facility or a skilled nursing facility. This includes transfers from nursing homes, long-term care facilities, and skilled nursing facilities where patients are receiving non-skilled level of care.

Outpatient: The patient was referred to the facility for outpatient or referenced diagnostic services by a physician of another healthcare facility where he or she is an outpatient.

- Emergency room

Inpatient: The patient was admitted to the facility for outpatient or referenced diagnostic services by the facility's emergency room physician.

Outpatient: The patient was referred to the facility for outpatient or referenced diagnostic services by the facility's emergency room physician.

- Court/law enforcement

Inpatient: The patient was admitted to the facility upon the direction of a court of law, or upon the request of a law enforcement agency representative.

Outpatient: The patient was referred to the facility upon the direction of a court of law, or upon the request of a law enforcement agency representative for outpatient or referenced diagnostic services.

- Newborns

  Normal Delivery: A baby delivered without complications

  Premature Delivery: A baby delivered with time and/or weight factors qualifying it for premature status

  Sick Baby: A baby delivered with medical complications, other than those relating to premature status

  Extramural Birth: A newborn delivered in a non-sterile environment

  Multiple Birth: Two or more babies delivered without complications

Special care unit: A medical care unit in which there is appropriate equipment and a concentration of physicians, nurses, and others who have special skills and experience to provide optimal medical care for critically ill patients or continuous care of patients in special diagnostic categories.

Standard deviation: The square root of the variance. The standard deviation is more easily interpretable as a measure of variation than the variance.

Stay outliers: *See* outliers

Stepdown unit: A unit used for cardiac patients for care between the cardiac intensive care unit and a general medical/surgical unit.

Stillbirth: The birth of a dead fetus.

Stillborn infant: A fetus, irrespective of its gestational age, that shows no evidence of life (such as heartbeats or respirations) after complete expulsion or extraction during childbirth. *Heartbeats* are to be distinguished from several transient cardiac contractions. *Respirations* are to be distinguished from fleeting respiratory efforts or gasps.

Surgery: Surgery includes incision, excision, amputation, introduction, endoscopy, suture and manipulation.

Surgical operation: One or more surgical procedures performed at one time for one patient via a common approach or for a common purpose.

Surgical procedure: Any single, separate, systematic process upon or within the body that can be complete in itself; is normally performed by a physician, dentist, or other licensed practitioner; can be performed either with or without instruments; and is performed to restore disunited or deficient parts, remove diseased or injured tissues, extract foreign matter, assist in obstetrical delivery, or aid in diagnosis.

Swing beds: Hospital-based acute care beds that may be used flexibly to serve as long-term care beds.

Table: An organized arrangement of data, usually appearing in columns and rows.

Tax Equity and Fiscal Responsibility Act (TEFRA): Federal legislation (enacted in 1983) designed to bring about prospective pricing Medicare in inpatient healthcare. Prospective pricing sets the fees for hospital care in advance of the care.

TEFRA: *See* Tax Equity and Fiscal Responsibility Act

Term neonate: Any neonate whose birth occurs from the beginning of the first day (267th day) of the 39th week, through the end of the last day of the 42nd week (294th day), following onset of the last menstrual period.

Tertiary care: Highly specialized care provided by specialists who use sophisticated technology and support services (such as a neurosurgeon, fertility specialist, or immunologist).

Third-party payer: A method of payment in which an entity other than the patient pays for services rendered to the patient. For example, an insurance company is a third party.

Total bed count days: The sum of inpatient bed count days for each of the days during a specified period of time.

Total billed charges: All charges for procedures and services rendered to the patient during a hospitalization or encounter.

Total inpatient service days: The sum of all inpatient service days for each of the days during a specified period of time.

Total length of stay: The sum of the days' stay of any group of inpatients discharged during a specified period of time. This is also known as *discharge days*.

Transfer: The movement of a patient from one treatment service or location to another. *See also* Intrahospital transfer

Trauma center: An emergency care center that is specially staffed and equipped to handle trauma patients. Most trauma centers are equipped with an air transport system.

Triage: The sorting of, and allocation of treatment to, patients. Triage is an early assessment that determines the urgency and priority for care and the appropriate source of care.

UB-92 Uniform Bill (HCFA 1450): A standardized uniform billing form required by federal authorities for Medicare claims. The UB-92 form is used as an industry standard.

UHDDS: *See* Uniform hospital discharge data set

Unbundling: A CPT coding method that uses several codes for each part of a procedure rather than the one comprehensive code that covers all the parts. The result is a higher reimbursement because the amount allowed under Medicare for the bundled (or single) amount is considerably lower than the sum of the amount for tests billed separately. Recently, Congress has passed legislation to fight healthcare fraud and abuse practices such as unbundling.

Uniform hospital discharge data set (UHDDS): A core set of data elements, adopted by the US Department of Health, Education, and Welfare in 1974, which are collected by hospitals on all discharges and all discharge abstract systems. The data set was revised by the National Committee on Vital and Health Statistics in 1984 and was implemented for federal health programs on January 1, 1986. Most hospitals collect and abstract this minimum data set.

Unique personal identifier: A unique number that the healthcare provider assigns to a patient. This number distinguishes the patient and his/her medical record from all others in the institution, assists in the retrieval of the record, and facilitates posting of payment.

Unique provider identification number (UPIN): A unique number assigned by the Health Care Financing Administration to identify physicians and suppliers who provide medical services or supplies to Medicare beneficiaries. UPINs for physicians, ordering and referring physicians, and suppliers are required when billing for Medicare services and are used to track payment and utilization information of individual physicians.

UPIN: *See* Unique provider identification number

Urgent admission: An admission in which the patient requires immediate attention for treatment of a physical or psychiatric problem.

Usual, customary, and reasonable charge: A charge for healthcare services based on a community norm or on a norm developed by a third party payer.

Utilization review: A review of the utilization of medical services based on the diagnosis, site, length of stay, and other factors in each case.

Variability: The difference between each score and every other score.

Variance: The sum of squared deviations of individual values from the mean divided by the sample size reduced by one. Variance provides a summary of the dispersion of individual observations around the mean.

Vocational rehabilitation: Evaluation and training aimed at assisting a person to enter or reenter the labor force.

Well newborn: A newborn born at term, under sterile conditions, with no diseases, conditions, disorders, syndromes, injuries, malformations, or defects diagnosed, and no operations other than routine circumcisions performed.

Workers compensation: Laws requiring employers to furnish care to employees injured on the job.

X-axis: On a graph, the horizontal axis where the independent variables are noted.

Y-axis: On a graph, the vertical axis that displays the frequency.

Years of schooling: The highest grade of schooling completed by the enrollee/patient. For children under the age of 18, the mother's highest grade of schooling completed should be obtained.

Index

Pages that include tables and figures are shown in *italic* type.

Adjusted hospital autopsy rate, 68–69
Adjusted member months, 84, 85
Agency for Health Care Administration, 2
AHCA. *See* Agency for Health Care
    Administration
ALOS. *See* Average length of stay
Alternative care settings, statistics computed for,
    83–91
Ambulatory care facilities, statistics maintained
    for, 87
American College of Surgeons, cancer annual
    report required by, 63
American Society of Addiction Medicine Patient
    Placement Criteria, 90
Anesthesia death rate, 62
Arithmetic average. *See* Mean
Autopsies, 65–72
Autopsy rate
    defined, 66
    gross, 66
    net, 66–67
Average daily census, 22–23
    for care unit, 23
    formulas for, 22, 23
    for newborns, 23
Average length of stay, 40–42, 116, *118–19*
    avoiding distortions in, 40
    formula for, 40
    for long-term care facilities, 87
    median used in, 40, 41
Average monthly census for long-term care facil-
    ities, 87
Average newborn length of stay, 40
    formula for, 42

Balanced Budget Act of 1997, 87
Bar graph, 108, *109*
Bed capacity. *See* Bed count
Bed complement. *See* Bed count
Bed count, 28–29
    change (expansion or reduction) in, 30–31
    defined, 28
Bed count days, 29
Bed days
    adjusted member months, 85
    calculated the same as hospital inpatient ser-
      vice day, 84
    commercial, 85
    defined, 84
    Medicaid, 86
    Medicare, 86
    unadjusted member months, 85
Bed occupancy ratio, 29–35
    defined, 29
    example of, 31
    formula for, 30
Bed turnover rate, 32–33
    direct and indirect formulas for, 32
Behavioral health settings, statistics for, 90

Calculation of transfers, 17–18
Cancer mortality rate, 62–63
Case-mix index statistical report, 117, *123*
Categorical data
    interval, 103
    nominal, 102
    ordinal, 102
    ranked, 102–3

Cells, table, *105*
Census
 average daily, 22–23
 average month, 87
 to calculate staff hours, 10, *12*
 complete master, 10–11
 daily, 12
 defined, 10
 example of, *11*
 time for taking, 10
 verifying, 18–19
Census day. *See* Inpatient service days
Central tendency, measures of, 5–7
Cesarean section rate
 example of, 51
 formula for, 50
Charts, patient, 76–79
 active/inactive, 76
 availability of, 76
 new, 76
 per FTE, ratio of, 79
 pulls of, 76
 requests for, 76
 responsibilities for maintaining, 76–79
Column headings, table, *105*
Complete master census, 10–11
Component parts of whole, pie graph to
 display, *111*
Computerization of statistics, 115–25
 spreadsheets for, 117, 124
 verifying reports from, 116–*23*
Continuous data, 103–4
Correspondence copying, costs for, 75

Data
 categorical, 102–3
 census, 9–25
 comparisons of, graphs to display, 104
 death rate, 60
 distortion of, tables to avoid, 104
 exact values of, tables to present, 104
 length of stay, 37–43
 numerical, 102, 103–4
 patient status, 9–25
 reported to state agencies, 2
 trends in, graphs to display, 104
 types of, 102–4
Data display, 104–11
 in graphs, 104, 107–11
 in tables, 104–7
Data presentation, 101–14
Dead on arrival (DOA) patients, 61
Death as type of discharge, 60

Death rates, 59–64
 anesthesia, 62
 avoiding rounding in computing, 47
 cancer, 62–63
 defined, 60
 fetal, 48–49, 61
 formula for, 60
 gross, 60
 guidelines for calculating, 60–61
 hospital, formula for, 60
 hospital, inclusions and exclusions for, 61
 infant, *46*–48
 maternal, 49–50, 61
 neonatal, *46*–48
 net, 61
 postoperative, 62
Descriptive statistics, 102
Dichotomous data, 102
Direct obstetric deaths, 49
Discharge days, 38
 difference between inpatient service days
  and, 39
 used in calculating average length of stay, 40
Discharge report, computerized, 116, *118–19*
Discrete data, 103

Emergency department
 calculating visits per month per 1,000 members to, 84, 86
 exclusion from hospital inpatient death rate of
  patients who die in, 61
Emergency department beds, 29, 29
Encounters per FTE per month, 77, 79

Fetal death rate, 61
 early, intermediate, and late deaths for, 48–49
 formula for, 48
Financial report, computerized statistical, 116,
 120–21
Frequency distribution
 normal distribution as, 97
 range as difference between largest and
  smallest values in, 94
 tables illustrating, 106–7
Full-time employees, ratios for calculating HIM,
 77, 79, 85

GAF scale, 90
Global assessment of functioning, 90
Graphs, 104, 107–11
 advantages of displaying data in, 104, 107

bar, 108, *109*
    basic form of, 108
    essential components in, 108
    histogram, 108, *109,* 110
    line, *110*
    pie, *111*
Gross autopsy rate, 66
Gross death rate, 60

HCUPnet, 2
Health information management department
    planning work space for, 79
    report of time allocation in, 77, *78*
    staffing levels in, ratios for determining, 77,
        79, 85
    statistics computed within, 73–81
HIM department. *See* Health information man-
    agement department
Histogram, 108
    example of, *109*
    rules for creating, 110
Hospital autopsies, 67–68
Hospital autopsy rate, adjusted
    example of, 68–69
    formula for, 68
Hospital death rate, 60, 61
Hospital fetal death, 48
Hospital inpatient autopsy, 67

In-and-out patients, 18
Indirect obstetric deaths, 49
Infant death defined, 46
Infant mortality rate, 46–48
    of developed nations for three time
        periods, *46*
    formula for, 47
Infection rate, 54
    postoperative, 54–55
Inpatient service days, 13–14
    bed days for MCOs calculated same as, 84
    calculation of, 16–18
    commercial, 84, 85
    defined, 13
    difference between discharge days and, 39
    example of, *16*
    Medicaid and Medicare, 84
    total, 14
Inpatient utilization for MCOs, bed days as
    measure of, 84–85
Interval data, 103
Intrahospital transfers, 11

Key, graph, 108, *109*

Leave of absence days, 42
Legend, graph, 108, *109*
Length of stay
    analysis of, 39
    average, 40–42, 87
    calculating, *38*
    defined, 38
    for mental health settings, 90
    newborn, average, 42
    total, 39
    uses of, 38
Length of stay data, 37–43
Line graph, *110*
Long-term care facilities
    example of statistical report for, *88*
    statistics used for, 87
Loose papers, measuring, 76
LOS. *See* Length of stay
LTCs. *See* Long-term care facilities

Managed care organizations, 84–86
Maternal death rate, 49–50, 61
    formula for, 49
    hospital, formula for, 50
    vital statistics, formula for, 50
MCOs. *See* Managed care organizations
Mean, 94
    defined, 6
    formula for, 6
    used in calculating average length of
        stay, 40, 41
Measures of central tendency, 5–7
    choice among, 7
Measures of variation, 93–99
Median
    defined, 6
    determining, 6–7
    used in calculating average length of
        stay, 40, 41
Medicaid
    bed days calculated for, 84
    bed days per 1,000 members for, 86
Medical transcription compensation, annual, 74
Medicare
    bed days calculated for, 84
    bed days per 1,000 members for, 86
    Part A services for skilled nursing
        facilities, 87
    percent of total discharges for, 2

Member months
  adjusted, 84, 85
  projected, 84
  unadjusted, 85
Mental health settings, statistics for, 90
Mode
  calculating, 7
  defined, 7
Morbidity, 54
Mortality rates, 59–64
  anesthesia, 62
  avoiding rounding in computing, 47
  cancer, 62–63
  defined, 60
  fetal, 48–49, 61
  formula for, 60
  gross, 60
  guidelines for calculating, 60–61
  hospital, formula for, 60
  hospital, inclusions and exclusions for, 61
  infant, *46–48*
  maternal, 49–50, 61
  neonatal, *46–48*
  net, 61
  postoperative, 62

Neonatal death, 46
Neonatal mortality rate
  formula for, 46
  vital statistics formula for, 47, *48*
Net autopsy rate, 66
Net death rate, 61
Newborn bassinet count, 28
Newborn bassinet occupancy ratio, 31
Nominal data, 102
Normal distribution, 97–98
  defined, 97
  visual inspection of data set as aid in
    discerning, 98
Number of patients remaining as census of
    patients at beginning of next day, 18
Numerical data
  continuous, 103–4
  discrete, 103

Observation, classifying beds for counts in, 29
Obstetrical and perinatal rates, 45–52
Optical disk storage, statistics for evaluating,
    79–80
Ordinal data, 102
"Other rates" formula, 55–56

Outliers
  comparing LOS data of facility to DRG LOS
    to find, 38
  example of, *97*
  mean as not sensitive to, 6

Patient care units
  census of, 10, 12
  intrahospital transfers for, 11
  studies of individual, 16
Patient census data, 9–25
Patient days. *See* Inpatient service days
Patient record processing, 76–79
Patients
  admitted and discharged on same day, census
    for, 18
  in-and-out, 18
  new versus established, 76
Per member per month (PMPM)
  estimating or budgeting, 84
  measured for resource allocations for
    MCOs, 84
Percentage
  defined, 3
  example of, *4*
  as type of ratio, 3–4
Pie graphs, *111*
PMPM. *See* Per member per month
Postneonatal death, 46
Postneonatal mortality rate, 47
Postoperative death rate, 62
Postoperative infection rate, 54–55
Projected member months measure, 84
Proportion
  defined, 3
  example of, *4*
  for nominal data, 102
  as type of ratio, 3
Providers per FTE per month, 79

Range as measure of variation, 94
Ranked data, 102–3
  example of, *103*
Rate
  calculating, 2
  defined, 4
  sample report using, *3*
  as type of ratio, 4–5
Ratio
  calculating, 2–3
  for determining HIM staffing levels, 77, 79

example of, *4*
newborn bassinet occupancy, 31
percentage as type of, 3–4
proportion as type of, 3
rate as type of, 4–5
Ratio data, 103
RBRVS. *See* Resource-based relative value
   system
Readmission rate statistical report, computerized,
   116, *122–23*
Recap as summary, 19
Recapitulation of census data, 18–19
   sample of, *19*
Record release, HIM staff time for, 77
Release of information
   centralized function for, 77
   cost breakdown for, 75
Reports. *See* Statistical reports
Resource-based relative value system, 87

Scale captions, graph, 108, *109*
SD. *See* Standard deviation
Skilled nursing facilities, per diem PPS for, 87
Source footnote
   graph, 108, *109*
   table, *105*
Spreadsheet software, 117, *124*
Staff workload and productivity, 74–75
Staffing hours, census to calculate, 10, *12*
Standard deviation, 96–97
   formula for, 96
   graph of, *97*
Statistical reports
   case-mix index, 117, *123*
   discharge, computerized, 116, *118–19*
   examples of, *5, 55*
   financial, computerized, 116, *120–21*
   readmission rate, computerized, 116, *122–23*
   spreadsheet software to create, 117, *124*
   verification of, 116–*23*
Statistics
   computed for alternative care settings, 83–91
   computed within HIM department, 73–81
   computerization of, 115–25
   descriptive, 102
Stillbirth, 49

Stubs and stub headings, table, *105*
Surgical operation, 54–55
Surgical procedure, 54

Tables
   advantages of, 104
   essential components of, 104–*5*
   examples of, *105*
   frequency distribution, 106–7
Telephone calls, HIM staff time for, 77
Time allocation in HIM department, reporting,
   76–78
Total inpatient service days, 14
Total length of stay, 39
Transfers, calculation of, 17–18
Trends
   graphs as revealing, 104
   time, line graphs to display, 110
Tumor registries, reporting to, 63

Unit medical transcription labor cost, 74–75
U.S. Agency for Healthcare Research and Quality (AHRQ), 2
Utilization management, review of LOS
   data in, 38

Variability as measure of spread, 94, 95
Variance
   budget, 96
   calculating, 96
   defined, 95
   formula for, 95
Variation, measures of, 93–99
   range as one of, 94
   variance as one of, 95–96
Vital statistics
   maternal mortality rate for, 50
   neonatal mortality rate for, 47, *48*

Work space for HIM department, statistics used
   for planning, 79